W9-BYI-799

The Technology of Orgasm

Johns
Hopkins
Studies
in the
History of
Technology

Merritt Roe Smith
Series Editor

The Technology of Orgasm

"Hysteria," the Vibrator, and Women's Sexual Satisfaction

Rachel P. Maines

The Johns Hopkins University Press
Baltimore & London

© 1999 The Johns Hopkins University Press
All rights reserved. Published 1999
Printed in the United States of America on acid-free paper
2 4 6 8 9 7 5 3 1

The Johns Hopkins University Press
2715 North Charles Street
Baltimore, Maryland 21218-4363
www.press.jhu.edu

Library of Congress Cataloging-in-Publication Data will be found
at the end of this book.
A catalog record for this book is available from the British Library.

ISBN 0-8018-5941-7

For my
mother,
who
taught me
that
intellectual
freedom
is worth
fighting for

Contents

Preface

When I was a teenager a family friend said I was the kind of kid who would come home from school and ask permission to undertake some risky venture by saying, "But Mummy! You have to let me! *Nobody's* doing it!" I've since decided that this is the judgment of my character I would want carved on my tombstone. The research I have set forth in this book is perhaps the most conspicuous example to date of my fascination with topics that nobody is doing.

When I first encountered vibrator advertisements in turn-of-the-century women's magazines in 1977, my reaction to their turgid prose was to assume that I simply had a dirty mind. I was, after all, twenty-seven years old, between marriages, a very angry feminist, and inclined to interpret everything I saw or read as some manifestation of the war between the sexes. A few years earlier, still in the throes of my first marriage, I had received Shere Hite's original questionnaire about women's sexuality; the prospect of responding to it was too depressing to contemplate. The same year I saw the vibrator ads, I read *The Hite Report*, which shed new light not only on my own experiences but on those of my women friends.

I am often asked, when I present papers at meetings, how I managed to find this esoteric topic. My usual reply is that I didn't—it found me. The advertisements I found fell on a prepared mind, or at the very least, on prepared hormones. Since graduating from college in 1971 (in classics, with emphasis on ancient science and technology), I had been interested in the textile arts, and I spent two years wondering naively why it was so difficult to find any serious, well-researched histories of the subject. In 1973 it dawned on me that this could only be because women did it. For me this was the "click" experience reported by so many feminists of the early seventies. All of a sudden I was fighting mad, determined to write serious needlework history come hell or high water. After all, nobody was doing it.[1]

Needlework proved to be an exciting and illuminating focus of research. It had a very rich primary literature plus a heritage of more artifacts than any one human being could live long enough to examine, but twenty years ago there were very few secondary sources and virtually no bibliographic access. Because my early interests had been in late nineteenth- and early twentieth-century American crochet, tatting, knitting, and embroidery, which were at that time poorly represented in the cataloged collections of large museums, there was nothing for it but to dive headfirst into the enormous unindexed sea of popular needlework publications, by the simple but laborious method of sitting down with whatever piles of them I could find and turning one page after another. In 1976 I was invited to present a paper on needlework history at a conference on women's history organized by Louise Tilly at the University of Michigan; it was later published as "American Needlework in Transition, 1880–1930."[2] As I doggedly turned the pages of *Modern Priscilla* and *Woman's Home Companion* in search of trends among the needlework patterns, my attention frequently strayed to the advertisements along the sides of the pages. It is a strong-minded historian indeed who can resist the lure of advertisements in historical periodicals; I am incapable of such iron self-discipline. Besides, I had an excuse: I was also looking for evidence that support from yarn and thread advertising was responsible for the large number of needlework periodicals published in the United States between 1880 and 1930.

When I saw vibrator advertisements as early as 1906 for equipment strongly resembling the devices now sold to women as masturbation aids, my first thought, as I said, was that this could not possibly be the purpose of the appliances sold in the pages of the *Companion*. The second thought was that 1906 was very early for any kind of home electrical appliance. Telling myself I'd never follow up on the topic, I made a few notes on the titles, issues, dates, and page numbers of needlework publications carrying vibrator advertisements. I showed a few of the ads to my feminist friends, who were, of course, delighted.

In the meantime my trip to Michigan to deliver my very first scholarly paper had borne unexpected fruit. A textile historian in the audience, Daryl Hafter of Eastern Michigan University, introduced herself and urged me to join the Society for the History of Technology and its subgroup, Women in Technological History (WITH). After one SHOT meeting I was convinced that it was time for graduate study in the history of technology. While I was in graduate school from 1979 to 1983, I continued to make notes on "sightings" of vibrator references while grinding away diligently at my dissertation on textile history. By this time it was clear to me that publishing my suspicions about the vibrator would torpedo my career; surely no one would ever again take me seriously as a scholar if I continued this line of research. On the other hand, nobody was doing it.

After I graduated from Carnegie-Mellon University, I spent three years as an assistant professor at Clarkson University in northern New York. As a part-timer, my teaching duties were light and I had plenty of time for research. While churning out articles on textile history, I began a little file on the vibrator and started looking for museum collections with relevant artifacts. According to curators Bernard Finn (electricity), Deborah Jean Warner (scientific instruments), and Audrey Davis (medicine) at the Smithsonian Institution, the nation's largest museum had no vibrators. Given that there were at least ten manufacturers of the devices in the United States in 1920, this was in itself somewhat odd. Chasing my topic through the various directories of museums and special collections, I wrote letters, including one to the Kinsey Institute, to which they replied with courtesy, promptness, and a very helpful bibliography, and one to an institution I had never heard of, the Bakken Library and Museum of Electricity in Life, in Minneapolis, Minnesota.

In writing to the Bakken Library I had carefully explained my research interests, describing the type of devices and documents I was seeking, and why. Throwing caution to the winds, in my concluding paragraph I commented that this was the first research I had ever done that appealed to both scholarly and prurient interest. Two weeks later I had a reply from the director that started, "Your letter appealed to our prurient interest . . ." Thus began a very fruitful research enterprise. The Bakken, founded by Earl Bakken of Medtronic, consists of a well-funded and scrupulously curated collection of historical medical instruments using electricity and an imposing library and archive of material relating to this topic. In the artifacts collection, the Bakken had eleven vibrators, listed in their catalog as "musculo-skeletal relaxation devices." A photograph of one of them is included in this book as figure 6. The library contained an overwhelming wealth of illustrations, texts, advertisements, and medical literature about my subject. I became a Bakken fellow for a week and spent five days wallowing in intellectual luxury. At the end of the week I made my first presentation on the vibrator to the staff and members of the Bakken and was asked to write a short article for the museum's newsletter, which became my first publication on the subject.

It was on this research trip that I first became aware that the subject of the vibrator polarizes audiences. The sympathetic good humor of the Bakken staff can best be illustrated by the following episode. The curator and I were down in collection storage examining the vibrator collection, photographing, weighing, and examining the objects. The curator, Al Kuhfeld, a conscientious scholar with a wry sense of humor, was taking the opportunity presented by the visiting scholar (me) to expand and update the information on his catalog cards. Since I had museum training, I was permitted to write (in pencil, of course) on the cards the new information, such as weight, measurements, number of vibratodes (attachments), and so on. We came to the artifact shown in figure 6, an early twentieth-century medical vibrator with a selection of about half a dozen vibratodes. I asked the curator if the device was still operational. Looking into the box, Al unerringly selected the most appropriate of the attachments, plugged the cord into a wall outlet, and flipped the switch. No response. Unplugging the device, he pulled a small screwdriver from his pocket, made several mysterious adjustments, and again plugged in the instrument, which then buzzed vigorously when turned on. After a moment's silent debate as to how this experiment should be performed, I placed the palm of my hand over the vibratode and mentally compared it with modern devices. Thanking Al, who began putting away the artifact, I wrote "runs" in the "remarks" section of the catalog card. The curator looked over my shoulder and nodded without comment. About half an hour later the museum's director came down and asked how we were getting along. I told him we had just plugged in one of the vibrators and tried it out. "And did it work?" he asked. "We don't know if it works," replied Al solemnly. "We only know that it runs."

At the seminar I presented at the Bakken, I saw for the first time the contrast between those who listen eagerly to my results, laughing at the inescapably humorous aspects, and those whose discomfort with the topic is expressed in a glazed look. Since then I have had numerous opportunities to observe these effects in audiences large and small. Groups consisting only of women simply laugh and ask questions. In mixed groups the women look uncomfortable and ask little, though they laugh just the same; they are aware that it is a major breach of etiquette to mention in mixed company the relative inefficiency of penetration as a means of producing female orgasm. The men are divided into laughter and blank stares: the former, I gather, are those for whom my research confirms that women are as sexual as they had always hoped, and the latter are those for whom it confirms that women are as sexual as they had always feared.

After my return from the Bakken, the Liberal Studies program at Clarkson wanted to publicize the then rare phenomenon of one of its members' receiving a fellowship, but there was concern about the reaction of the rest of the faculty (primarily engineers and scientists) to my subject matter. The issue was resolved by placing a notice in the faculty newsletter that I had "received a grant-in-aid . . . from the Bakken Library of Electricity in Life in Minneapolis, Minnesota. She will use the grant to study the impact of small electric appliances in the home."[3]

Shortly after completing my brief article for the Bakken newsletter, I began to receive invitations to present papers on the vibrator to university audiences. At this point I discovered what I should have realized all along: that some people, most of them male, take my findings personally and resent them as an implied criticism. One of my first academic venues for this topic was a long-established institution housed in ponderous, ivy-covered stone buildings. About eight people attended the seminar I spoke at, with the male faculty arranged on one side of the table and the women faculty and graduate students on the other side. After my presentation, one tenured senior professor (wearing the obligatory herringbone tweed jacket) said he was not entirely convinced by my argument, since the sexual experience of women using vibrators and their predecessors was "not the real thing." While I was collecting my wits to formulate some sort of response to this fundamental misunderstanding, one of the women graduate students rescued me. "Don't you see, Dr. So-and-So? Most of the time, it's better than the real thing." Her female colleagues nodded solemnly, and Dr. So-and-So subsided. This was clearly not what he wanted to hear. I have since encountered this objection in many forms, of which the most straightforward, as I recall, was the complaint, "But if what you're saying is true, then women don't need men!" The only possible reply is that if orgasm is the only issue, men don't need women either.

I also gave a presentation at a medical school in Canada, a prospect that terrified me, since I would have to tell my hair-raising story to physicians. To my surprise, they reacted with the same polarization I had observed elsewhere, with one relatively minor difference: before the presentation one doctor simply refused to believe that I was actually going to talk about vibrators. My paper had been given some innocuous title like "Physical Therapies from Aretaeus to Freud," but one of his students told him what was really going to be discussed. When he saw me in the hall he said, "You wouldn't believe what people told me you're going to talk about!" When I replied that the rumors, however vicious, were probably true, he vigorously denied that it was possible. "But she said you were going to talk about vibrators!" When I confirmed that this was indeed my topic, he was aghast, but he showed up anyway. After the talk he complained that no doctor could now get away with such goings-on as I described, which of course is true. One of his colleagues jeered at this objection: "Oh, come off it. You're just sorry you missed all this." Needless to say, the audience roared. A historian commented to me afterward that he had noted the blank stares of those who had asked no questions. "There's a lot of peer pressure not to seem uptight in those situations," he said. "They just smile and think of the queen."

In June 1986, right after the publication of my first article on the vibrator in the Bakken newsletter, I lost my job at Clarkson University. I had been teaching in the School of Management, and before that in the Liberal Studies program. One afternoon I picked up my mail and found a photocopied list of new office assignments. My name was not on it. Inquiries to the dean revealed that I no longer had a job at Clarkson. There seemed to be several reasons, among them that my intellectual interests simply did not fit into the School of Management, but there were two other complaints: first, it was feared that alumni would stop giving money to the school if it was discovered that a member of its faculty was doing research on vibrators, and second, that my very high energy level "wasn't compatible with the rest of the faculty." Since I had only a part-time position, there was nothing for it but to pack my books and go.

I had already been doing some contract cataloging work for a museum near the university, so when I left Clarkson I expanded my client base and became the owner of a business that provides cataloging, inventory, and research services to museums and archives. Meanwhile I continued to make presentations and give papers on the vibrator, including one at Cornell University near my new home in Ithaca, New York, and another at the Society for the History of Technology's annual meeting in October 1986. At this latter, my audience appeared to be struggling desperately to keep a straight face, probably out of a misguided respect for my scholarly dignity, until I called the vibrator a "capital-labor substitution innovation." This produced a hearty guffaw from the Smithsonian's curator of scientific instruments, Deborah Jean Warner, after which others seemed to realize it was all right to laugh. One of the questions raised at this meeting was asked by a well-known Darwin scholar, who pointed out that doctors who failed to recognize the orgasm in their patients must never have seen one in their wives.

By far the most entertaining of my adventures with vibrator historiography, however, was the brouhaha occasioned by my 1989 article in *Technology and Society*, a publication of the Institute of Electrical and Electronics Engineers (IEEE): "Socially Camouflaged Technologies: The Case of the Electromechanical Vibrator." Early in 1988 I had noticed a call for papers for a special issue of *Technology and Society*, under the editorship of Robert Whelchel, with eminent electrical historian James Brittain as guest editor. I cobbled together a brief discussion of the social camouflage aspect of my research and sent it in; the article went through the usual referee process and was accepted with revisions. The only hint of possible trouble was a letter from Brittain that closed by saying my article was to be a kind of test of IEEE publication policy, as they had not published an article like mine "since they began in 1884."

The article was published in July, when many professors and engineers are on vacation. In September I received a telephone call from Bob Whelchel. The Technical Advisory Board (TAB) of IEEE was threatening to withdraw the publication charter of *Technology and Society* on the grounds that since there couldn't possibly be anyone named Rachel

Maines who had actually written this article, it must be some sort of elaborate practical joke on the part of the co-editors. It could not, according to the TAB, have been refereed, and the references must all have been faked. The nine-page article had fifty-one footnotes to more than 160 sources, some of them in Latin and Greek. As one TAB member expressed it, "It read like a parody of an IEEE article. It contained dozens and dozens of obsolete references." Whelchel and Brittain were preparing for an inquiry at the November 1989 TAB meeting, at which they would be required to show proof of my existence (!), evidence that Maines and Associates was a respectable business establishment, and proof that the article had been refereed. Others were busily verifying the existence of my references.[4]

Shortly before the November meeting, I received another call, this time from a reporter for IEEE *Spectrum*, a newspaper that goes out to all 350,000 members of IEEE. The October issue had a half-page article on the foofaraw on the Technical Advisory Board, including a quotation from one member who thought I should have used radar detection devices in automobiles as my example of a socially camouflaged technology. He also considered my article as written more "to titillate than to enlighten," apparently rejecting the possibility that both could occur simultaneously. At the meeting, cooler heads prevailed: referee reports were shown, a letter from my colleagues in the Society for the History of Technology was produced, and the antivibrator faction was made to realize that the IEEE was in danger of making itself a laughingstock. Letters in later issues of *Spectrum* all expressed the view that it was about time for the IEEE to take a courageous look at some new issues. I was told that subscriptions to *Technology and Society* went up as a result of the controversy, illustrating yet again that efforts at censorship simply provide valuable publicity for what they attempt to suppress.

Acknowledgments

Like all hardworking historians, I have more intellectual debts than I can remember or repay. Over the decade I spent writing this book, my two most important supports have been my husband, Garrel Pottinger, and my friend Karen Reeds. Although neither resorted to nagging, both made it clear that they would accept no excuses for my failing to complete the book.

I have, of course, taxed the patience and ingenuity of any number of librarians, archivists, and curators. Among these, I owe the greatest debt to Elizabeth Ihrig and Albert Kuhfeld of the Bakken Library and Museum of Electricity in Life, in Minneapolis, Minnesota. Without the material the Bakken staff provided while I was a fellow there in the summer of 1985, this project would not have amounted to much more than a speculative article or two. The support of the Bakken Fellowship program enabled me to make the discoveries in the primary sources that convinced me I was on solid historical ground.

The libraries of Cornell University, especially the History of Science collection, have proved invaluable, as have the collections of the National Library of Medicine, the Library of Congress, the New York Public Library, the Charcot Library of the Salpêtrière in Paris, the Saratoga County Historical Society in Ballston Spa, New York, the Center for the History of American Needlework, the Kinsey Institute at Indiana University, and the Saratoga Room collection on hydrotherapy and balneology at the Saratoga Springs (New York) Public Library.

As sources of inspiration and guidance I must acknowledge Shere Hite of Hite Research, Joel Tarr of Carnegie-Mellon University, and my former students at Clarkson University in Potsdam, New York, especially my Great Ideas in Western Culture students Marianne Incerpi and Gary Cassier. James Glynn III of Comtech, Incorporated, provided valuable insights into why so many people find this subject disturbing. Participants in seminars and meeting sessions asked important questions that needed answers at the 1986 meeting of the Society for the History of Technology at Queens University in Kingston, Ontario, the University of Ottawa Hannah Lectures in the History of Medicine series, and the Cornell University Humanities Colloquium. Joani Blank of Down There Press and Good Vibrations in California provided useful material on early vibrators and has been a consistent source of encouragement, as was Dell Williams of Eve's Garden in New York City.

I owe a debt of gratitude to Robert J. Whelchel of Tri-State University and James Brittain of the Georgia Institute of Technology for their courageous decision to publish my article "Socially Camouflaged Technologies: The Case of the Electromechanical Vibrator," in the July 1989 issue of the IEEE's *Technology and Society*.

My editors and reader at the Johns Hopkins University Press deserve credit for their courage and sensitivity, as well: series editor Merritt Roe Smith, history editor Bob Brugger, reader Ruth Schwartz Cowan, Sarah Cline of the acquisitions department, marketing manager Hilary Reeves, and production editor Kimberly Johnson. Alice Bennett provided the kind of meticulous copyediting which all authors should have and aren't capable of doing for themselves.

Gretchen Aguiar put a mind-numbingly long bibliography into a format that made it possible to find the references I needed when I needed them. Last but definitely not least, I doubt I would have found the courage to persist in my eccentricities, especially this one, had not my best friends cheered me on: Catherine Gatto Oliver, Judith Ruszkowski, Karen La Monica, and of course my mother, Natalie L. M. Petesch.

The Technology of Orgasm

1

The Job Nobody Wanted

In 1653 Pieter van Foreest, called Alemarianus Petrus Forestus, published a medical compendium titled *Observationem et Curationem Medicinalium ac Chirurgicarum Opera Omnia*, with a chapter on the diseases of women. For the affliction commonly called hysteria (literally, "womb disease") and known in his volume as *praefocatio matricis* or "suffocation of the mother," the physician advised as follows:

> When these symptoms indicate, we think it necessary to ask a midwife to assist, so that she can massage the genitalia with one finger inside, using oil of lilies, musk root, crocus, or [something] similar. And in this way the afflicted woman can be aroused to the paroxysm. This kind of stimulation with the finger is recommended by Galen and Avicenna, among others, most especially for widows, those who live chaste lives, and female religious, as Gradus [Ferrari da Gradi] proposes; it is less often recommended for very young women, public women, or married women, for whom it is a better remedy to engage in intercourse with their spouses.[1]

As Forestus suggests here, in the Western medical tradition genital massage to orgasm by a physician or midwife was a standard treatment for hysteria, an ailment considered common and chronic in women. Descriptions of this treatment appear in the Hippocratic corpus, the works of Celsus in the first century A.D., those of Aretaeus, Soranus, and Galen in the second century, that of Äetius and Moschion in the sixth century, the anonymous eighth- or ninth-century work *Liber de Muliebria*, the writings of Rhazes and Avicenna in the following century, of Ferrari da Gradi in the fifteenth century, of Paracelsus and Paré in the sixteenth, of Burton, Claudini, Harvey, Highmore, Rodrigues de Castro, Zacuto, and Horst in the seventeenth, of Mandeville, Boerhaave, and Cullen in the eighteenth, and in the works of numerous nineteenth-century authors including Pinel, Gall, Tripier, and Briquet.[2] Given the ubiquity of these descriptions in the medical literature, it is surprising that the character and purpose of these massage treatments for hysteria and related disorders have received little attention from historians.

The authors listed above, and others in the history of Western medicine, describe a medical treatment for a complaint that is no longer defined as a disease but that from at the least the fourth century B.C. until the American Psychiatric Association dropped the term in 1952, was known mainly as hysteria.[3] This purported disease and its sister ailments displayed a symptomatology consistent with the normal functioning of female sexuality, for which relief, not surprisingly, was obtained through orgasm, either through intercourse in the marriage bed or by means of massage on the physician's table. I shall place this disease paradigm in the context of androcentric definitions of sexuality, which explain both why such treatments were socially and ethically permissible for doctors and why women required them. Androcentric views of sexuality, and their implications for women and for the physicians who treated them, shaped the development not only of the concept of female sexual pathologies but also of the instruments designed to cope with them.

Technology tells us much about the social construction of the tasks and roles it is designed to implement. Although massage instrumentation has had many medical uses in history, I am concerned here only with its role in the treatment of a certain class of "women's complaints." The vibrator and its predecessors in the history of medical massage technologies are the means by which I shall examine three themes: androcentric definitions of sexuality and the construction of ideal female sexuality to fit them; the reduction of female sexual behavior outside the androcentric standard to disease paradigms requiring treatment; and the means by which physicians legitimated and justified the clinical production of orgasm in women as a treatment for these disorders. In evaluating these technologies, the perspective of gender is significant: for example, men typically react to figure 1 by wincing, and women laugh. Clearly, where technologies impinge on the body, especially its sexual organs, the sex of the body matters.

When the vibrator emerged as an electromechanical medical instrument at the end of the nineteenth century, it evolved from previous massage technologies in response to demand from physicians for more rapid and efficient physical therapies, particularly for hysteria. Massage to orgasm of female patients was a staple of medical practice among some (but certainly not all) Western physicians from the time of Hippocrates until the 1920s, and mechanizing this task significantly increased the number of patients a doctor could treat in a working day. Doctors were a male elite with control of their working lives and instrumentation, and efficiency gains in the medical production of orgasm for payment could increase income. Physicians had both the means and the motivation to mechanize.

The demand for treatment had two sources: the proscription on female masturbation as unchaste and possibly unhealthful, and the failure of androcentrically defined sexuality to produce orgasm regularly in most women.[4] Thus the symptoms defined until 1952 as hysteria, as well as some of those associated with chlorosis and neurasthenia, may have been at least in large part the normal functioning of women's sexuality in a patriarchal social context that did not recognize its essential difference from male sexuality, with its traditional emphasis on coitus. The historically androcentric and pro-natal model of healthy, "normal" heterosexuality is penetration of the vagina by the penis to male orgasm. It has been clinically noted in many periods that this behavioral framework fails to consistently produce orgasm in more than half of the female population.[5]

Because the androcentric model of sexuality was thought necessary to the pro-natal and patriarchal institution of marriage and had been defended and justified by leaders of the Western medical establishment in all centuries at least since the time of Hippocrates, marriage did not always "cure" the "disease" represented by the ordinary and uncomfortably persistent functioning of women's sexuality outside the dominant sexual paradigm. This relegated the task of relieving the symptoms of female arousal to medical treatment, which defined female orgasm under clinical conditions as the crisis of an illness, the "hysterical paroxysm." In

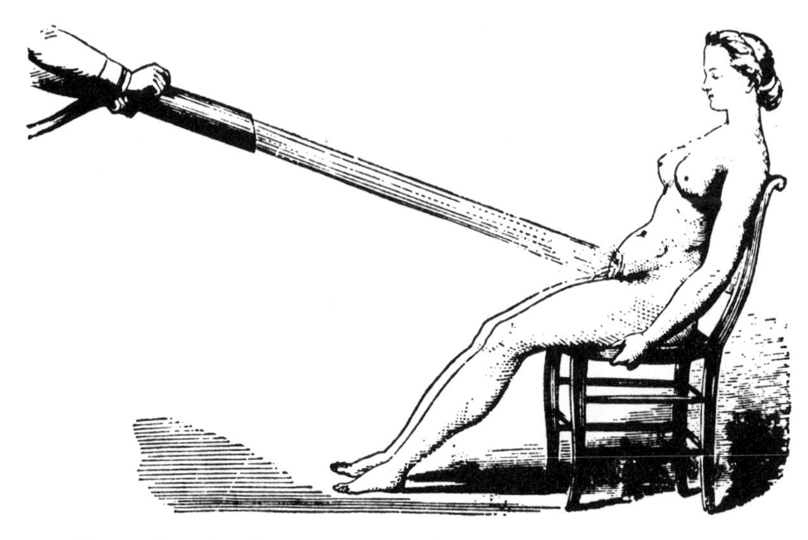

Fig. 1. French pelvic douche of about 1860 from Fleury, reproduced from Siegfried Giedion, *Mechanization Takes Command* (New York: Oxford University Press, 1948).

effect, doctors inherited the task of producing orgasm in women because it was a job nobody else wanted.

There is no evidence that male physicians enjoyed providing pelvic massage treatments. On the contrary, this male elite sought every opportunity to substitute other devices for their fingers, such as the attentions of a husband, the hands of a midwife, or the business end of some tireless and impersonal mechanism.[6] This last, the capital-labor substitution option, reduced the time it took physicians to produce results from up to an hour to about ten minutes.[7] Like many husbands, doctors were reluctant to inconvenience themselves in performing what was, after all, a routine chore. The job required skill and attention; Nathaniel Highmore noted in 1660 that it was difficult to learn to produce orgasm by vulvular massage. He said that the technique "is not unlike that game of boys in which they try to rub their stomachs with one hand and pat their heads with the other."[8] At the same time, hysterical women represented a large and lucrative market for physicians. These patients neither recovered nor died of their condition but continued to require regular treatment.

Russell Thacher Trall and John Butler, in the late nineteenth century, estimated that as many as three-quarters of the female population were "out of health," and that this group constituted America's single largest market for therapeutic services.[9] Furthermore, orgasmic treatment could have done few patients any harm, whether they were sick or well, thus contrasting favorably with such "heroic" nineteenth-century therapies as clitoridectomy to prevent masturbation.[10] It is certainly not necessary to perceive the recipients of orgasmic therapy as victims: some of them almost certainly must have known what was really going on.[11]

The Androcentric Model of Sexuality

The androcentric definition of sex as an activity recognizes three essential steps: preparation for penetration ("foreplay"), penetration, and male orgasm. Sexual activity that does not involve at least the last two has not been popularly or medically (and for that matter legally) regarded as "the real thing."[12] The female is expected to reach orgasm during coitus, but if she does not, the legitimacy of the act as "real sex" is not thereby diminished.[13] That more than half of all women, possibly more than 70 percent, do not regularly reach orgasm by means of penetration alone has been brought to our attention by researchers such as Alfred Kinsey and Shere Hite, but the fact was known, if not well publicized, in previous centuries.[14] This majority of women have traditionally been defined as abnormal or "frigid," somehow derelict in their duty to reinforce the androcentric model of satisfactory sex.[15] These women may constitute most of the hysterics of history, whose numbers make plausible Thomas Sydenham's argument in the seventeenth century that hysteria was "the most common of all diseases except fevers."[16] It also explains the contention of nineteenth-century doctors that hysteria was pandemic in their time.[17] When marital sex was unsatisfying and masturbation discouraged or forbidden, female sexuality, I suggest, asserted itself through one of the few acceptable outlets: the symptoms of the hysteroneurasthenic disorders.

Historically, women have been discouraged from masturbating on the grounds that this practice would impair their health, and most men before this century (even to this day, some would argue) have not understood that penetration alone is sexually satisfying to only a minority of women. Even those husbands and lovers who may have known did not always want to take the trouble to provide the additional stimulation necessary to produce female orgasm.[18] Medical authorities as recently as the 1970s assured men that a woman who did not reach orgasm during heterosexual coitus was flawed or suffering from some physical or psychological impairment. The fault must surely be hers, since it was literally unimaginable that any flaw could be discovered in the penetration hypothesis.[19] If the penis did not represent the ultimate weapon in sexual warfare, claims to male superiority would rest entirely on the statistically greater potential of the male biceps and deltoid muscles, which did not in themselves seem equal to the task of sustaining patriarchy in Western civilization.

Female orgasm and the means of producing it were and are anomalous from a biological as well as a political and philosophical point of view. Its lack of correlation with fertility and conception remains counterintuitive even—perhaps especially—in an age of greater scientific understanding of human reproduction. The biological function of the female orgasm is controversial.[20] In both the recent and the distant past, it seemed only reasonable to assume a priori that men and women would be sexually gratified by the same act of penetration to male orgasm that made conception possible. That stimulation of the external genitalia in women should be necessary in most cases remains unexplained.[21] As a historian, I would not presume to speculate on the physiological and evolutionary questions raised by this issue. I look forward with interest to the results of current inquiries by evolutionary biologists, reproductive physiologists, and physical anthropologists.

The question of female orgasm in history is deeply clouded by the androcentricity of existing sources. Medical authors, for example, have addressed female orgasm mainly from a prescriptive viewpoint; popular writers only occasionally mention it at all.[22] Before the middle of this century, even in literature, references to female orgasm are conspicuous by their absence, even from works purportedly built around sexual subject matter.[23] In the development of Western medical thought on the subject of sexuality, it has been thought both reasonable and necessary to the social support of the male ego either that female orgasm be treated as a by-product of male orgasm or that its existence or significance be denied entirely. Historically, both strategies have been used, but there has also been a persistent undercurrent of recognition that the androcentric model of sexuality does not adequately represent the experience of women.[24]

Confusing the medical discussions of these issues, as Thomas Laqueur has pointed out, is the failure of the Western tradition until the eighteenth century to develop a complete and meaningful vocabulary of female anatomy. The vulva, labia, and clitoris were not consistently distinguished from the vagina, nor the vagina from the uterus. Thus it is difficult, in reading the premodern literature of gynecology, to decipher treatment descriptions in which the female genitalia are undifferentiated. Female sexuality is often referred to in masculine terms, such as the references to the secretions of the Bartholin glands as "semen" or "seed." Thomas Laqueur says that physicians writing of anatomy "saw no need to develop a precise vocabulary of genital anatomy because if the female body was a less hot, less perfect, and hence less patent version of the canonical body, the distinct organic, much less genital, landmarks mattered far less than the metaphysical hierarchies they illustrated."[25]

Hysteria as a Disease Paradigm

I intend to sketch here the contours of male medical and technological response to discontinuities between male and female experiences of sexuality through the social construction of disease paradigms. Situated in the vulnerable center of every past and present heterosexual relationship, the potentially destabilizing issues of orgasmic mutuality have historically been shifted to a neutral and sanitized ground on which female sexuality was represented as a pathology and female orgasm, redefined as the crisis of a disease, was produced clinically as legitimate therapy. This interpretation obviated the need to question either the exalted status of the penis or the efficacy of coitus as a stimulus to female orgasm. Furthermore, it required no adjustment of attitude or skills by male sex partners. What Foucault calls the "hystericization of women's bodies" protected and reinforced androcentric definitions of sexual fulfillment.[26]

Part of my argument here rests on the vague and sexually focused character of hysteria as defined by ancient, medieval, Renaissance, and modern medical authorities before Sigmund Freud. Many of its classic symptoms are those of chronic arousal: anxiety, sleeplessness, irritability, nervousness, erotic fantasy, sensations of heaviness in the abdomen, lower pelvic edema, and vaginal lubrication.[27] The paralytic states described by Freud and a few others are rarely mentioned by physicians before the late nineteenth century.[28] During the syncope some hysterics were observed to experience, as Franz Josef Gall pointed out in the second decade of the nineteenth century and A.F.A. King some seventy years later, the subject's apparent loss of consciousness was associated with flushing of the skin, "voluptuous sensations," and embarrassment and confusion after recovery from a very brief loss of control—usually less than a minute.[29] That hysterics did not become incontinent during their "spells" as epileptics did, and apparently felt much better afterward, led some physicians to suspect their patients of malingering. Doctors pointed out that epileptics often injured themselves when they fell, but that hysterics rarely did so.[30] I do not mean that all women diagnosed as hysterical were cases of sexual (or rather orgasmic) deprivation; some were no doubt afflicted with other mental or physical ailments whose symptoms overlapped significantly with the hysterical disease paradigm. Joan Brumberg has pointed out, for example, that in the nineteenth century many physicians believed that anorexia in young girls was a hysterical disorder.[31] But the sheer number of hysterics before the middle of this century, and their virtual disappearance from history thereafter, suggests it is perceptions of the pathological character of these women's behavior that have altered, not the behavior itself.[32]

The partial or complete loss of consciousness—or more properly, of reactivity to outside stimuli—was variously interpreted and described over time. Aretaeus, like Plato, believed that the inflamed and disconnected uterus was suffocating or choking the patient, a theme dwelt on at considerable length in late classical, medieval, and Renaissance medical writings. The uterus, engorged with unexpended "seed" (*semen* in Latin), was thought to be in revolt against sexual deprivation. The cure, consistent with the humoral theory popularized by Galen, was to coax the organ back into its normal position in the pelvis and to cause the expulsion of the excess fluids.[33] When the patient was single, a widow, unhappily married, or a nun, the cure was effected by vigorous horseback exercise, by movement of the pelvis in a swing, rocking chair, or carriage, or by massage of the vulva by a physician or midwife, as described by

Forestus in the paragraph quoted above. Single women of marriageable age who experienced hysterical symptoms were usually urged to marry and, as Ambroise Paré expressed it in the sixteenth century, "bee strongly encountered by their husbands."[34] Masturbation by the patient herself was not recommended as a treatment for hysteria until the early twentieth century, and then only rarely.[35] If hysteria was for the most part no more than the normal functioning of female sexuality, the inducement of the crisis of the disease, called the "hysterical paroxysm," would in fact have provided the kind of temporary relief physicians described. Only a handful of the medical authorities who advocated female genital massage as a treatment for hysteria, however, acknowledged that the crisis so produced was an orgasm.[36]

In the nineteenth century, as noted by Peter Gay and others, the received wisdom that women required sexual gratification for health came into conflict with newer ideas regarding the intrinsic purity of womanhood. A not uncommon resolution of the conflict of medical philosophies over women's sexuality was the compromise position that women ardently desired maternity, not orgasm.[37] This pro-natal hypothesis not only preserved the illusion of women's spiritual superiority while explaining their observed sexual behavior but also reinforced the ethic of coitus in the female-supine position as a divinely ordained norm. As Gay rightly points out, this proposition also protected the male ego and the androcentric model of sexuality.[38]

Freudian interpretations after 1900 presupposed sexual drives in women, placing these in a new kind of androcentric moralism, that of psychopathology, that was to persist into our own time. In the new paradigm, hysteria was caused not by sexual deprivation but by childhood experiences, and it could be manifested in propensities to masturbation and to "frigidity" in the context of penetration.[39] These two "symptoms" were also evidence, in the Freudian view, of female sexual development arrested at a juvenile level. The mystique of penetration thus could remain unchallenged even as the theoretical ground shifted under the medical and sexual issues. Real women, according to Freudian theory as well as earlier authorities, experienced mature sexual gratification as a result of vaginal penetration to male orgasm and accepted no substitutes for the "real thing." The role of the clitoris in arousal to orgasm was systematically misunderstood by many physicians, since its function contradicted the androcentric principle that only an erect penis could provide sexual satisfaction to a healthy, normal adult female.[40] That this principle relegated the experience of two-thirds to three-quarters of the female population to a pathological condition was not perceived as a problem.[41]

This androcentric focus, in fact, in many cases effectively camouflaged the sexual character of medical massage treatments. Since no penetration was involved, believers in the hypothesis that only penetration was sexually gratifying to women could argue that nothing sexual could be occurring when their patients experienced the hysterical paroxysm during treatment. Even the nineteenth-century physicians who excoriated the speculum for its allegedly stimulating effects and questioned internal manual massage saw nothing immoral or unethical in external massage of the vulva and clitoris with a jet of water or with mechanical or electromechanical apparatus.[42] Freudian and later interpretations of hysteria and masturbation helped undermine this camouflage, and when the vibrator, used in physicians' offices since the 1880s, began to appear in erotic films in the 1920s, the illusion of a clinical process distinct from sexuality and orgasm could not be sustained.[43]

In the evidence I present here on the histories of sexuality and medical massage in hysteria, it is important to stress that the voices of women are seldom heard. It is a rare person of either sex who sees fit to leave a record even of his or her most orthodox procreative marital sexuality, let alone of experiences with masturbation. In most historical times and places in Western culture, a woman's keeping such a record would have been unspeakably shocking and unchaste; its discovery might have subjected her to severe social sanctions. Even historians of male heterosexuality struggle with the lack of primary material; what remains may be fragmentary, or revised by embarrassed heirs or publishers. Historians must rely on largely prescriptive androcentric and pro-natal medical sources for much of our information on humanity's most intimate activities, because we have nothing else. Nearly all my sources relate to members of the middle to upper classes of white women in Europe and the United States, and it would be presumptuous to generalize from them to other cultures, classes, or races.[44]

The Evolution of the Technology

The electromechanical vibrator, invented in the 1880s by a British physician, represented the last of a long series of solutions to a problem that had plagued medical practitioners since antiquity: effective therapeutic massage that neither fatigued the therapist nor demanded skills that were difficult and time-consuming to acquire. Mechanized speed and efficiency improved clinical productivity, especially in the treatment of chronic patients like hysterics, who usually received a series of treatments over time. Among conditions for which massage was indicated in Western medical traditions, one of the most persistent challenges to physicians' skills and patience as physical therapists was hysteria in women. This was one of the most frequently diagnosed diseases in history until the American Psychiatric Association officially removed the hysteroneurasthenic disorders from the canon of modern disease paradigms in 1952.[45]

Mechanized treatments for hysteria offered a number of benefits to users of the technology—doctors, patients, and patients' husbands. Not only did the clinical production of the "hysterical paroxysm" provide a palliative for female complaints and make patients feel better, at least temporarily, it resolved the dissonance of reality with the androcentric sexual model. And since mechanical and electromechanical devices could produce multiple orgasms in women in a relatively short period, innovations in the instrumentation of massage permitted women a richer exploration of their physiological powers.[46] Although manual, hydriatic, and steam-powered mechanical massage offered some of these advantages, the electromechanical vibrator was less fatiguing and required less skill than manual massage, was less capital intensive than either hydriatic or steam-powered technologies, and was more reliable, portable, and decentralizing than any previous physical therapy for hysteria. Within fifteen years of the introduction of the first Weiss model in the late 1880s, more than a dozen manufacturers were producing both battery-powered vibrators and models operated with line electricity.[47] Some physicians even had vibratory "operating theaters" (see fig. 7).

Although manufacturers and users of massage technologies have called the instruments by a variety of names, here I use a relatively consistent nomenclature designed to emphasize the differences among various types of massage apparatus. First, a true vibrator is a mechanical or electromechanical device imparting a rapid and rhythmic pressure through a contoured working surface, which is generally mounted at a right angle to the handle. The applicators usually take the form of a set of interchangeable rubber vibratodes contoured to the anatomical surfaces they are intended to address. Vibrating dildos, a variant of the vibrator, are usually straight-shafted and are designed for vaginal or anal insertion.[48] A massager, as the term is used here, is a device with flat or dished working surfaces designed mainly for manipulating the skeletal muscles. All of these are distinct from the electrodes used in electrotherapy, which imparted a mild electrical shock to the tissues they were applied to and thus are technologically related to the vibrator only in a collateral way.

As we have seen, manual massage of the vulva as a treatment for hysteria or "suffocation of the mother" is continually attested in Western medicine from antiquity through the Middle Ages, Renaissance, and Reformation and well into the modern era. I have already quoted Forestus's 1653 description of the basic manual technique, which seems to have varied little over time except in the types of lubricating oils. Medical descriptions of this procedure were more or less explicit in their instructions to doctors, according to the temperament of the author. A few, like Forestus and his contemporary Abraham Zacuto (1575–1642), expressed reservations about the propriety of massaging the female genitalia and proposed delegating the job to a midwife.[49] The main difficulties for physicians, however, were the skills required to properly locate the intensity of massage for each patient and the stamina to sustain the treatment long enough to produce results.[50] Technological solutions to both problems seem to have been attempted fairly early in the form of hydrotherapeutic approaches and crude instruments like rocking chairs, swings, and vehicles that bounced the patient rhythmically on her pelvis.

We know very little about the ancient use of hydrotherapy in hysteria. Baths, however, particularly those built over hot springs, have a long history of association with sensuality and sexuality. Saint Jerome (340?–420), for example, admonished women, especially young women, to avoid bathing, since it "stirred up passions better left alone."[51] Female masturbation in this context typically requires that the water be in motion, preferably under some kind of pressure or gravitational force, so still bathing of the type depicted in medieval scenes of "stews" (see fig.

8, in chapter 4) would probably not have been effective.[52] Roman bath configurations usually included piped water that could have been used in this way, but evidence is lacking.[53] It is probable that many women in history independently discovered that water in motion had a stimulating effect, but these discoveries are unlikely to be documented except in the form of the vague prohibitions on sensual indulgence in the bath by medical and religious writers. By the late eighteenth century, specialized hydrotherapeutic appliances had been developed for female disorders and were in use in some European and British spas. There are few detailed descriptions or illustrations of these devices. Tobias Smollett remarked in 1752 on the number of hydriatic devices at Bath that were specially designed for women.[54] Women represented a majority of the market for hydriatic massage in Britain from at least Smollett's time. Many spas had special "female departments," and at least in America, women were often the owners, co-owners, or resident physicians of hydriatic establishments.[55]

The "social lion" of water cure establishments was the douche, or high-pressure shower, which was widely used in women's disorders as a local stimulant to the pelvic region (fig. 1). Henri Scoutetten, a French physician writing in 1843, described the popularity of the cold-water douche with his female patients as follows:

> The first impression produced by the jet of water is painful, but soon the effect of the pressure [*percussion*], the reaction of the organism to the cold, which causes the skin to flush, and the reestablishment of equilibrium all create for many persons so agreeable a sensation that it is necessary to take precautions that they [*elles*] do not go beyond the prescribed time, which is usually four or five minutes. After the douche, the patient dries herself off, refastens her corset, and returns with a brisk step to her room.[56]

The chief drawbacks of hydriatic massage for physicians, other than its apparently excessive allure for patients, were its capital intensiveness and its centralizing character: the equipment was expensive and required a semipermanent installation with a source of water, preferably heated.[57] Although some American manufacturers made efforts to popularize hydrotherapeutic equipment for clinics and even affluent private homes, the apparatus was prohibitively expensive and could not easily

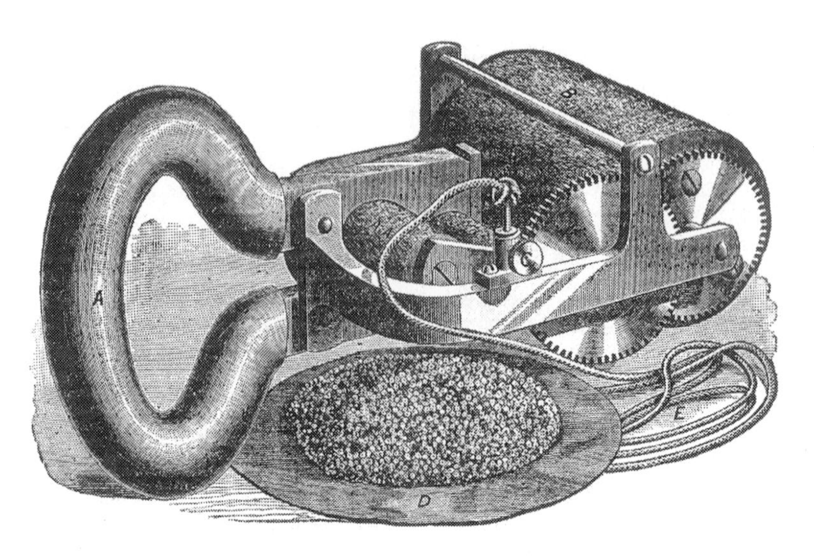

Fig. 2. Butler's Electro-massage Machine, from *Dr. John Butler's Electro-massage Machine* (New York: Butler Electro-massage, 1888).

be retrofitted to existing plumbing.[58] Patient and doctor thus had to travel to hydrotherapeutic treatment sites, where transportation, spa fees, lodging, and meals restricted the market to the upper middle class and above.[59]

Spas also represented the market for many early efforts to mechanize massage. Most had manual physical therapy equipment, such as muscle beaters, in their clinical arsenals, and when Gustaf Zander's (1835–1920) "Swedish Movement" machinery became available in the mid-nineteenth century, prosperous hydriatic establishments added this technology as well.[60] A clockwork "percuteur," essentially a wind-up vibrator, was also available to both spas and physicians before 1870 (see fig. 18, chapter 4). The percuteur, however, was underpowered for massage purposes and had a distressing tendency to run down before treatment was complete. Roller-type devices were sold in the popular market (fig. 2) that combined massage with electrotherapy; these were sold to both sexes and were touted as especially effective for renewing sexual vigor in men.[61]

In 1869 and 1872 an American physician, George Taylor, patented steam-powered massage and vibratory apparatus, some of it designed for female disorders. His principal markets were spas and physicians with a sufficiently large physical therapy practice to justify the expense of a large, heavy, and cumbersome instrument. Taylor warns physicians that treatment of female pelvic complaints with the "Manipulator" should be supervised to prevent overindulgence. One of his devices (fig. 3) featured a padded table with a cutout for the lower abdomen, in which a vibrating sphere, driven by a steam engine, massaged the pelvic area.[62]

Swedish efforts to produce a mechanical massage device on the principles of Zander's movement machinery produced results by the late 1870s, but the first electromechanical vibrator to be internationally marketed to physicians was the British model built by Weiss. Designed by the physician Joseph Mortimer Granville, the device patented in the early 1880s was battery powered and, like the modern version, equipped with several interchangeable vibratodes. Mortimer Granville, however, was firmly opposed to the use of his device for treating women, especially hysterics, and advised its application only to the male skeletal muscles.[63] Few physicians in the United States or elsewhere seem to have shared his compunction on this point, except for those who noted with concern that the devices induced uterine contractions in pregnant women.[64]

By 1900 a wide range of vibratory apparatus was available to physicians, from low-priced foot-powered models to the Cadillac of vibrators, the Chattanooga (fig. 4), which cost $200 plus freight charges in 1904.[65] Monell reported in 1902 that more than a dozen medical vibratory devices were available for examination at the Paris Exposition of 1900.[66]

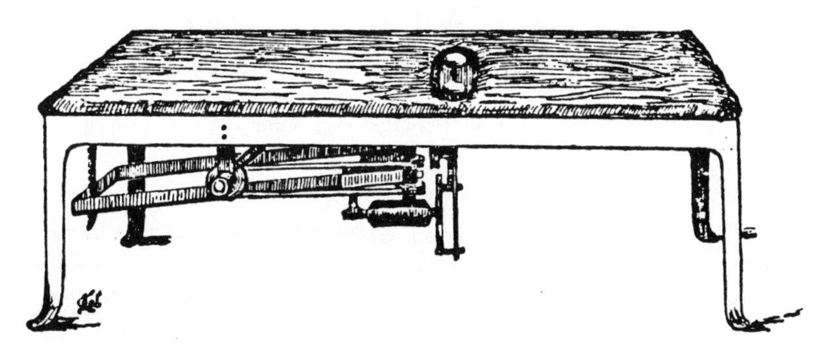

FIG. 3. The patient interface for George Taylor's steam-powered "Manipulator" of the late 1860s, from George Henry Taylor, *Pelvic and Hernial Therapeutics* (New York: J. B. Alden, 1885).

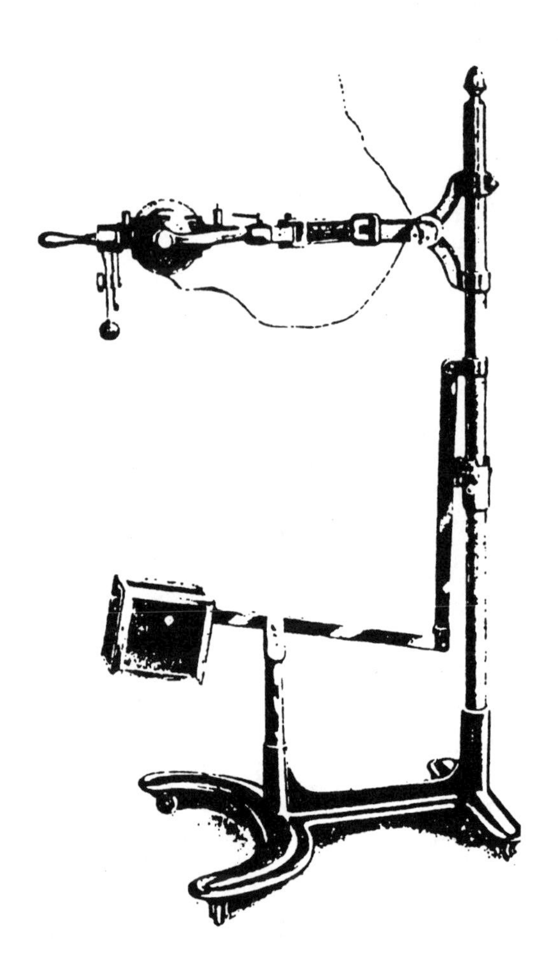

Fig. 4. The Chattanooga Vibrator, sold to physicians for about $200 in 1900. From *The Chattanooga Vibrator* (Chattanooga, Tenn., Vibrator Instrument Company, [ca. 1904]), cover.

Mary L. H. Arnold Snow, writing for a readership of physicians in 1904, discusses in some detail about twice this number, including musical vibro-massage, counterweighted types, tissue oscillators, vibratory forks, hand- or foot-powered massage devices, simple concussors and muscle beaters, vibratiles (vibrating wire apparatus), combination cautery and pneumatic equipment with vibratory massage attachments, and vibrators powered by air pressure, water turbines, gas engines, batteries, and street current through lamp-socket plugs.[67] These models, starting at $15 and ranging to the top of the line mentioned above, delivered vibrations to the patient at rates of one to seven thousand pulses per minute. Some were floor-standing machines on rollers, some were portable, and others could

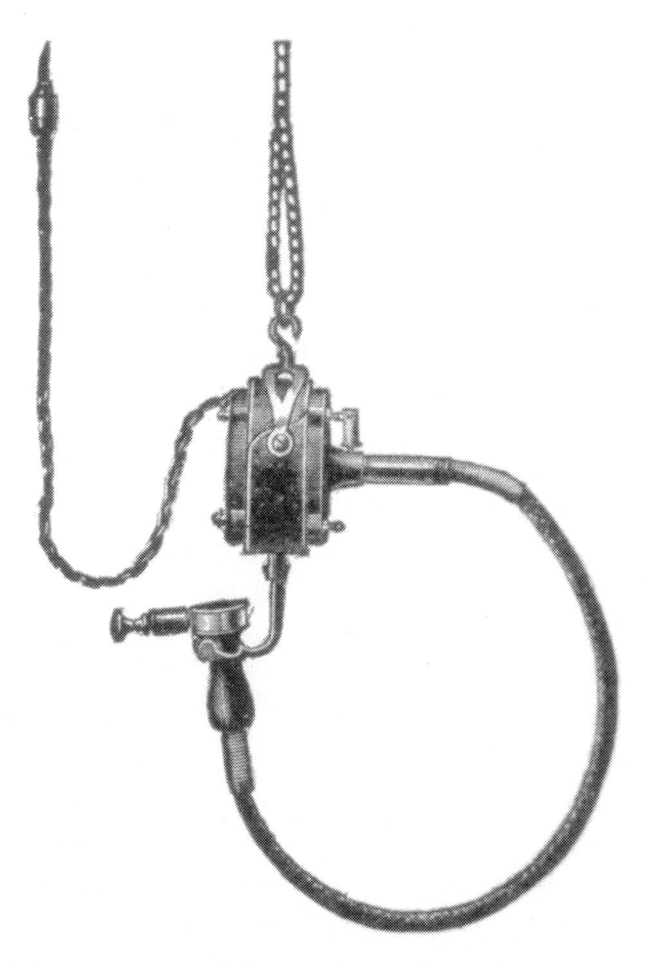

FIG. 5. "Hanging type of Carpenter vibrator," from Mary Lydia Hastings Arnold Snow, *Mechanical Vibration and Its Therapeutic Application* (New York: Scientific Authors, 1904).

be suspended from the ceiling of the clinic like impact wrenches in a modern garage (fig. 5).

Articles and textbooks on vibratory massage technique at the turn of this century praised the machine's versatility for treating nearly all diseases in both sexes and its savings in the physician's time and labor, especially in gynecological massage.[68] By 1905 convenient portable models

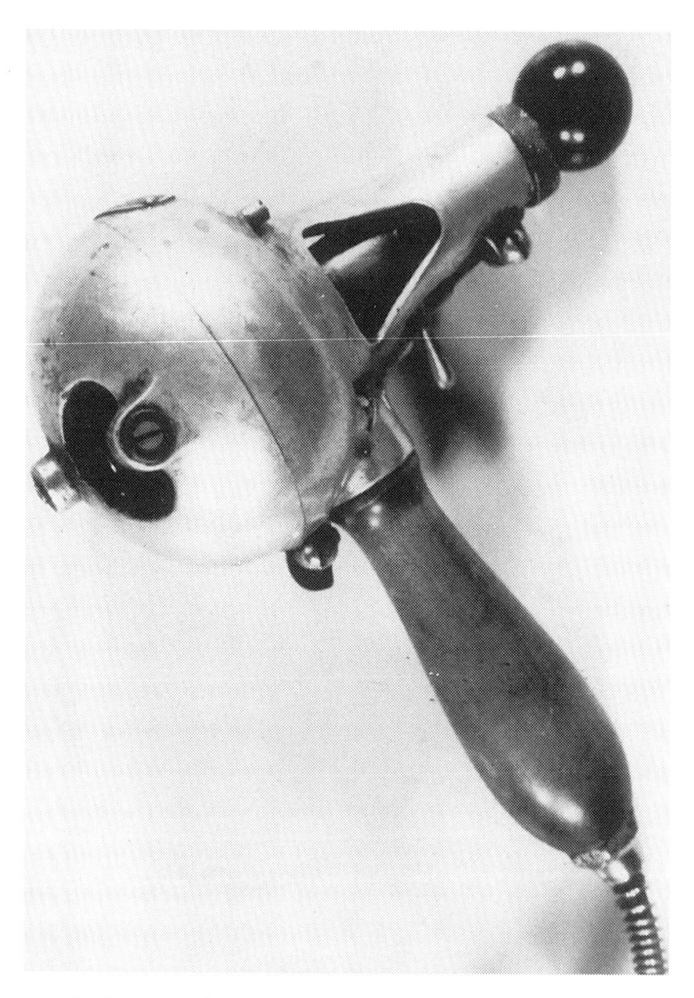

Fig. 6. Early twentieth-century medical vibrator at the Bakken Library and Museum of Electricity in Life.

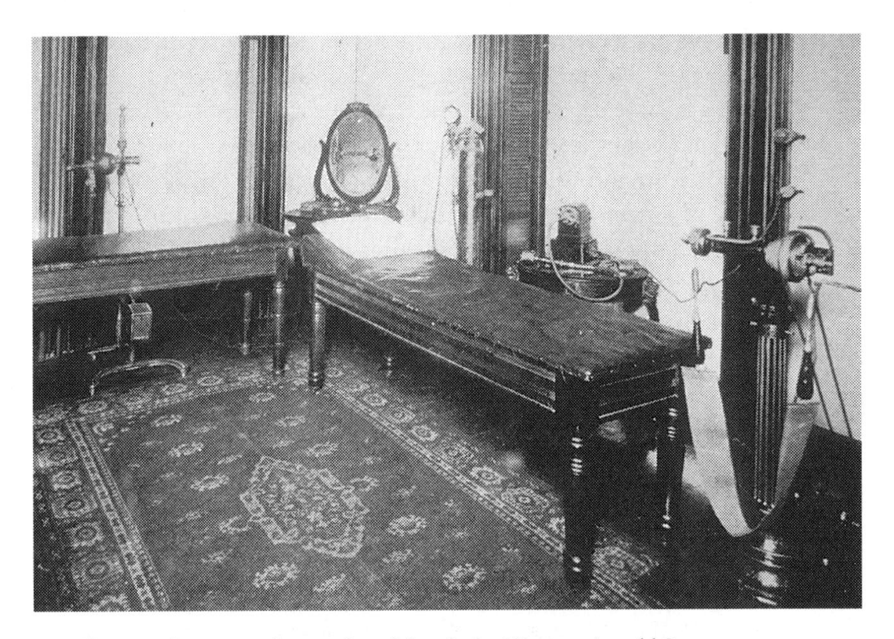

Fig. 7. Operating theater, from Mary Lydia Hastings Arnold Snow, *Mechanical Vibration and Its Therapeutic Application* (New York: Scientific Authors, 1904).

were available, with impressive arrays of vibratodes, permitting use on house calls (fig. 6).[69]

In the first two decades of this century, the vibrator began to be marketed as a home appliance through advertising in such periodicals as *Needlecraft*, *Home Needlework Journal*, *Modern Women*, *Hearst's*, *McClure's*, *Woman's Home Companion*, and *Modern Priscilla*. The device was marketed mainly to women as a health and relaxation aid, in ambiguous phrases such as "all the pleasures of youth . . . will throb within you."[70] When marketed to men, vibrators were recommended as gifts for women that would benefit the male givers by restoring bright eyes and pink cheeks to their female consorts.[71] A variety of models were available at all price ranges and with various types of power, including electricity, foot pedal, and water.[72] An especially versatile vibrator line was illustrated in the Sears, Roebuck and Company *Electrical Goods* catalog for 1918. Here an advertisement headed "Aids That Every Woman Appreciates" shows a vibrator attachment for a home motor that also drove attachments for churning, mixing, beating, grinding, buffing, and operating a fan (see fig. 24, chapter 4).[73]

The social camouflage of the vibrator as a home and professional medical instrument seems to have remained more or less intact until the end of the 1920s, when the true vibrator (but not massagers or electrotherapeutic devices) gradually disappeared both from doctors' offices and from the respectable household press. This may have been the result of greater understanding of women's sexuality by physicians, the appearance of vibrators in stag films in the twenties, or both. Electrical trade journals of the period did not mention vibrators or report statistics on their sale as they did for other medical appliances.[74]

When the vibrator reemerged during the 1960s, it was no longer a medical instrument; it had been democratized to consumers to such an extent that by the seventies it was openly marketed as a sex aid.[75] Its efficacy in producing orgasm in women became an explicit selling point in the consumer market. The women's movement completed what had begun with the introduction of the electromechanical vibrator into the home: it put into the hands of women themselves the job nobody else wanted.

2

Female Sexuality as Hysterical Pathology

Most of us are familiar with the current popular meanings of the word "hysterical." Applied to a person, it means "upset to the point of irrationality"; applied to a situation, it means "very funny." The usage has shifted from the technical designation of a disease paradigm to much more general references to uncontrolled, usually frivolous, emotions.

This development, occurring primarily since World War II, is only the latest in two and a half millennia of kaleidoscopic refocusing on feelings and behavior usually constructed as quintessentially feminine.[1] The term "hysteria" comes from a Greek word meaning simply "that which proceeds from the uterus." "Hysterical" thus combines in its connotations the pejorative elements of femininity and of the irrational; there is no analogous word "testerical" to describe, for example, male sports fans' behavior during the Super Bowl.[2] Hysteria as a disease paradigm has been variously constructed over time by physicians and their patients, but at all times and places it has retained its focus on the intrinsic pathology of the feminine, even (or perhaps especially) when applied to males. Assumptions of sexual pathology, of the innate "wrongness" or "otherness" of women familiar to readers of Aristotle, form the set of basic elements—the colored glass in the kaleidoscope—that are recombined by the mechanism of social and technological change. Mainstream Western medical theory and practice have shifted these central assumptions—altering their relations, changing perspectives on them, finding new language and new conceptual frameworks in which to interpret them, but have rarely questioned the androcentric ideology that embedded these concepts in Western thought. Although physicians in the nineteenth century believed hysteria had reached epidemic proportions, the disease paradigm was by no means a Victorian invention; its antecedents were far more venerable and deeply entrenched.

In this chapter I intend to show how the disease paradigm of hysteria and its "sister" disorders in the Western medical tradition have functioned as conceptual catchalls for reconciling observed and imagined differences between an idealized androcentric sexuality and what women actually experienced. I must beg readers' indulgence for what will of necessity be a confusing journey through the definition of hysteria; my sources contradict themselves, confuse cause and effect, or change their minds from one century or one decade to the next about the direction of causality. I have already stated that these hypotheses about the now-banished disease paradigm of hysteria had only a few common elements. Ilsa Veith's magisterial 1965 work *Hysteria: The History of a Disease* provides a comprehensive and well-documented overview of the evolution of a disease paradigm that had, at the time of the book's publication, only recently passed into history. Veith says that "hysteria . . . has adapted its symptoms to the ideas and mores current in each society; yet its predispositions and its basic features have remained more or less unchanged." Edward Shorter, too, has written on the "blizzard of symptoms" that have at various times and places been incorporated into the concept of hysteria.[3]

Hysteria in Antiquity and the Middle Ages

Ancient physicians from the fifth century B.C. until well after the end of the classical era, whether Greek, Roman, or Egyptian, were in fairly close agreement on what hysteria was, and their definition persisted in several important strands of Western medical thought until Jean-Martin Charcot and Sigmund Freud swept all before them at the end of the nineteenth century.[4] Freud's view was in fact so persuasive that historians since his time have been inclined to impose his reinterpretation of the hysteroneurasthenic disorders on the preceding 2,500 years of clinical observation.[5] I shall have more to say of this at the end of this chapter.

Hysteria was a set of symptoms that varied greatly between individuals (and their physicians), including but not limited to fainting (syncope), edema or hyperemia (congestion caused by fluid retention, either localized or general), nervousness, insomnia, sensations of heaviness in the abdomen, muscle spasms, shortness of breath, loss of appetite for food or for sex with the approved male partner, and sometimes a tendency to cause trouble for others, particularly members of the patient's immediate family.[6] The disorder was thought to be a consequence of lack of sufficient sexual intercourse, deficiency of sexual gratification, or both. Physicians committed to the androcentric model of sexuality were inclined to conflate these two etiologies and to prescribe treatment accordingly, as we shall see. Jean-Michel Oughourlian reports some of the observed characteristics of the hysterical paroxysm in clinically precise yet somehow unilluminating terms: "What is a hysterical crisis? On the clinical level, excito-motor paroxysmic accidents accompanied by convulsions and crises of inhibition with loss of consciousness, lethargy, or catalepsy have been recognized for four thousand years."[7]

Hysteria appears in the medical corpus as early as 2000 B.C. in Egypt, but it was not until the time of Hippocrates in the fifth century B.C. that the Western clinical definition of the disorder began to take shape. In the Hippocratic corpus, hysteria is a disease of the womb, treatable with exercise and massage.[8] Plato's reference to hysteria as a disease caused by the uterus, "an animal inside an animal," is well known. By the time of Celsus and Soranus in the first century A.D., genital massage and exercise, usually passive, were standard prescriptions for hysteria.[9] Soranus advocated manipulating the groin and pubic area: "We . . . moisten these parts freely with sweet oil, keeping it up for some time." He suggested baths and swinging in a hammock as adjunct therapies for chronic cases.[10] Aretaeus Cappodox, writing a century later on mania as a chronic disease, discusses the causes of the ailment, asserting that "women . . . become affected with mania from want of purgation of the system, when the uterus has attained its full development."[11] Caelius Aurelianus, writing in the third century A.D., recapitulates the symptomatologies of Hippocrates, Soranus, and Aretaeus.

Galen (ca. A.D. 129–200), the physician's physician for centuries after his death, described hysteria as a uterine disease caused by sexual deprivation, to which passionate women were particularly susceptible. This theme of female sexuality as pathology was to reappear in various forms in later centuries. He describes in detail a genital massage therapy, resulting in contractions and the release of a fluid from the vagina, after which the patient was relieved of her symptoms. His account is literally the classic description of massage therapy for hysteria, which was to be repeated almost verbatim in later texts and to be regarded as therapeutic gospel in some medical circles until the end of the nineteenth century. Rudolph Siegel's translation has often been quoted: "Following the warmth of the remedies and arising from the touch of the genital organs required by the treatment, there followed twitchings accompanied at the same time by pain and pleasure after which she emitted turbid and abundant sperm. From that time on she was free of all the evil she felt."[12]

Later writers echoed Galen's advice, sometimes adding clinical observations of their own. Äetius of Amida (502–75), described in his "Tetrabiblion" a hysterical paroxysm characterized by uterine contractions, muscular spasm in the entire body, and discharge of fluid from the vagina.[13] As in both earlier and later accounts, this event is described as bringing the patient symptomatic relief. Moschion's (Mustio, Muscione) *Gynaecia* of the same century makes similar, if less graphic, references to the paroxysmal therapeutic result of manual friction to the vulva.[14]

Medieval texts rarely called the disorder in question "hysteria," although it retained its character as a disease of the uterus. Much of this literature recalled Plato's account of the uterus wandering around the body, causing problems as it went, particularly strangulation as it allegedly crawled up into the chest and windpipe.[15] The panting and shortness of breath associated with the hysterical paroxysm, and eventually the disease itself, came to be called the "suffocation of the uterus" or the "suffocation of the mother." The medieval corpus attributed to Trotula says this ailment is due to "the retaining of blood or of corrupt and venomous uterine humors that should be purged in the same way that men are purged of seed that comes from their testicles next to the penis." Both sexes were thought to suffer illnesses from retention of this seed.[16]

The literature of midwifery, some of which was written by women, paralleled an elite body of medical works by men in the Middle Ages. One of the male luminaries of this period was Rhazes (865?–925?), an influential Arabic physician. His work on massage of the vulva in hysteria was widely cited and quoted by Western physicians. Danielle Jacquart and Claude Thomasset summarize the views of Avicenna (980–1037) on hysteria. Marriage was the best remedy, but if all else failed, masturbation to orgasm was indicated: "According to Avicenna the cure was efficacious only if the sensations of coitus that is, pleasure and pain, were felt. Medieval doctors generally omitted to refer to this aspect of the treatment when recommending recourse to manipulation; yet it was evident that female sexual discharge accompanied orgasm."[17] One might infer from this passage that Avicenna or his colleagues might have occasionally advocated masturbation by the woman herself. This is not the case. In the *Canon* he warns of women's resorting to "rubbing, among other women" as a possible consequence of unsatisfying intercourse; it is clearly not intended as advice on recommended practice for women.[18] The privilege (or drudgery) of such "rubbing" was reserved for husbands, doctors, and midwives.

Arnaldus of Villanova (ca. 1235–ca. 1311) recommended that the discharge of offending fluids be achieved in widows and nuns by friction and internal massage with what Veith calls "irritating suppositories inserted in the vagina," consistent with the theory of readjusting the balance of humors.[19] The thirteenth-century document by Pseudo-Albertus provides the usual background to the etiology of the disease in sexual deprivation and makes the mandatory reference to Galen's massage techniques. Marriage and intercourse were, as usual, prescribed. According to Helen Rodnite Lemay, the Italian Anthonius Guaynerius (Antonio Guainerio, d. 1440) discussed the disease in substantially the same way; Lemay says of his account that "among the indications of suffocation caused by retention of sperm is the absence of male companionship in the life of a woman who was accustomed to it." One of the treatments was "to anoint the mouth of the vulva with different odoriferous materials, for which the prescription is also included, and to rub it into the neck of the womb as well. The rubbing, which should be done with the midwife's finger, will cause the womb to expel the sperm or corrupt humors and free the patient from disease."[20]

Giovanni Matteo Ferrari da Gradi (d. 1472), the "Gradus" of the Forestus quotation in chapter 1, wrote a commentary and explication of Rhazes' medical practice for the Europeans of his day called *Practica, seu Commentaria in Nonum Rasis ad Almansorem*. He essentially repeats the therapeutic advice already familiar by his time, adding that the chest should be rubbed and covered closely with large cupping glasses, after which "the midwife would be instructed to use sweet-smelling oil on her finger and move it well in a circle inside the vulva."[21] Ferrari da Gradi goes on to mention that marriage and childbearing sometimes cure, but only if the woman experiences "maior delectatio" (greater pleasure) in conjugal sex, and how in successful treatment, the patient experiences "simul . . . delectatio & dolor" (pleasure and pain at the same time). This too echoes earlier descriptions. He describes the release of fluid after the paroxysm and says that retention of these fluids by the chaste and widowed causes hysteria.

A transitional figure between the Middle Ages and the Renaissance was Paracelsus (1493–1541), whose real name was Philippus Theophrastus Bombastus von Hohenheim. A famous, or perhaps notorious, physician and alchemist, in "On the Diseases That Deprive Man of His Reason" he wrote of hysteria, which he also called "chorea lascivia." The crisis of this disease, he asserted, was characterized by contractions of the uterus and vagina.[22]

Hysteria in Renaissance Medicine

The tradition of treating hysteria by evacuating fluids insalubriously retained is continued in the sixteenth and seventeenth centuries. The famous surgeon Ambroise Paré (1517?–1590) wrote some lively accounts both of hysteria and of its proposed treatments:

> Those who are free'd from the fit of the suffocation of the womb either by nature or by art, in a short time their color commeth in to their faces by little and little, and the whole beginneth to wax strong, and the teeth, that were set, and closed fast together, begin (the jaws being loosed) to open and unclose again, and lastly som moisture floweth from the secret parts with a certain tickling pleasure; but in some women, as in those especially in whom

the neck of the womb is tickled with the Midwive's finger, in stead of that moisture com's thick and gross seed, which moisture or seed when it is fallen, the womb being before as it were rageing, is restored unto its own proper nature and place, and by little and little all symptoms vanish away.[23]

Marriage and intercourse were thought to be curative in many cases. When hysteria was diagnosed, "If she be married, let her forthwith use copulation, and bee strongly encountered by her husband, for there is no remedy more present than this." If this remedy was unavailable, "Let the mydwife annoint her fingers with *oleum nardinum* or moschetalinum, or of cloves, or else of spike mixed with musk, ambergreese, civet and other sweet powders, and with these let her rub or tickle the top of the neck of the wombe which toucheth the inner orifice."[24]

Audrey Eccles quotes Riverius (Lazare Rivière, 1589–1655) as follows:

Womb-Furie is a sort of madness, arising from a vehement and unbridled desire of Carnal Imbracement, which desire disthrones the Rational Facul[ty] so far, that the Patient utters wanton and lascivious Speeches . . . [Although it mainly affects virgins and young widows,] it may also betide married women, that have impotent Husbands, or such as they do not much affect, whereby their seminary vessels are not sufficiently disburthened . . . [If marriage fails as a remedy] some advise that the Genital Parts should be by a cunning Midwife so handled and rubbed, so as to cause an Evacuation of the over-abounding Sperm.[25]

According to Eccles, Riverius's assessment of the situation was typical of his time. Quoting Nicholas Culpeper, she asserts that "most authors were persuaded that the best way to bring down the uterus and discharge the seed was by sexual intercourse" and goes on to describe the standard method involving the midwife's finger dipped in aromatic oil. "Not unnaturally," she says, "there was some doubt whether this course of action was quite unexceptionable, morally speaking, a scruple which Culpeper considered a foolish Popish superstition."[26]

Robert Burton (1577–1640) discusses a symptomatology cognate with hysteria under the heading "Maid's, Nun's and Widow's Melancholy." Like most of his predecessors, he recommends marriage as a cure.

After general discussion of diet and environmental issues, he tells us that "the best and surest remedy of all is to see them well placed and married to good husbands in due time, hence these tears, that's the primary cause, and this is the ready cure, to give them content to their desires."[27] Burton opposed celibacy for nuns and priests, partly on the grounds that, in his opinion, it encouraged masturbation. Giulio Cesare Claudini, writing in 1607, recommended massage as an alternative to marital intercourse in the treatment of hysterics, observing that "limited counterirritation applied to the lower parts, with which friction of the parts at the same time, painful binding, and an abundance of lubricating oil are regarded as appropriate."[28]

Concerns about the mental state of women religious was not unusual in the seventeenth century. G. Rattray Taylor comments on concerns with hysteria and supposed demonic possession among nuns, remarking on the similarity of symptoms between hysterical and sexual manifestations. He notes that "hysterical seizures usually bear a close relationship to the unconscious fantasy: in particular, women sometimes exhibit convulsive body movements, or become rigid, with the body arched so that the pudenda are thrust forward as in coitus."[29] Taylor interprets this behavior in the context of the androcentric model and assumes that it is driven by a repressed desire for penetration.

Michael MacDonald observes somewhat patronizingly that seventeenth-century physicians perceived a correlation between women's medical conditions and their psychological states and that "they tried to persuade their fellow practitioners and the literate public that an ailment they called 'suffocation of the mother' was widespread." Hysterical symptoms were caused by "the alleged propensity of the uterus to become a vagabond, leaving its proper place in the womb [*sic*] and wandering into the upper parts, near the passionate heart."[30] As we have seen, this disease paradigm was well entrenched in the medical community long before the seventeenth century.

Abraham Zacuto (1575–1642), called Zacutus Lusitanus, endorsed in his *Praxis Medica Admiranda* of 1637 the standard medical view that marriage was best for hysterics but that friction of the vulva by a physician or midwife could be employed if the preferred treatment failed. He first describes a case of marriage as a successful therapy, in terms that must have been reassuring to those committed to the androcentric model of sexuality:

> Nor should you wonder at all these things which are natural to women, and are particularly to be expected of the condition of virgins; because of retention of the sexual fluid, the heart and surrounding areas are enveloped in a morbid and moist exudation: this is especially true of the more lascivious females, inclined to venery, passionate women who are most eager to experience physical pleasure; if she is of this type she cannot ever be relieved by any aid except that of her parents, who are advised to find her a husband. Having done so, the man's strong and vigorous intercourse alleviated the frenzy. She married an energetic young man, who, having discharged his marital responsibilities with vigor, she took to this with enthusiasm; under this appropriate treatment she flourished, revived, bloomed with the rosy shade of well-being, and was entirely restored to health.[31]

He goes on, however to describe a "virginella" for whom it was necessary to use a pessary made from cyclamen, onion, garlic, and ox gall, "from the motion of which and the excitement and heat it aroused in the private parts, a copious quantity of sexual fluid was emitted and was visible after the fury of the attack had subsided." Zacuto expresses concern about whether "God-fearing physicians" ought really to perform such procedures and concludes that they are acceptable when women are in danger of death from hysteria. But he also notes that not all of his colleagues concur: "As to whether to draw this harmful fluid out of the uterus by exciting and rubbing the private parts, Raphael Moxius and Carrerius disagree most articulately."

Nicolaas Fonteyn (Nicolaus Fontanus, fl. 1630) made a colorful presentation in 1652 of the views of his time on this subject, in the characteristically florid and inconsistent English of seventeenth-century vernacular medical documents:

> Wives are more healthfull then Widowes, or Virgins, because they are refreshed with the mans seed, and ejaculate their own, which being excluded, the cause of the evill is taken away. This is evident from the words of *Hippocrates*, who adviseth young Maids to marrie, when they are thus troubled;

> that women have stones [testicles; i.e., ovaries or glands] and seed, no true Anatomist will denie; the womans seed, I confess, in regard of the small quantitie of heat, is more imperfect then the seed of the mans, yet is it most absolute in itselfe, and fit for Generation. Another cause also may be added, besides that which is alledged from *Hippocrates*, namely, that married women by lying with their husbands, doe loosen the passages of the seed, and so the Courses come down more easily throw them; Now in Virgins it falls out otherwise, because the bloud is stopped by the constipation and obstruction of the veines, and being stopped putrifies, from which putrifaction grosse vapours doe arise, and from thence heavinesse of minde, and dulnesse of spirit, a benummednesse of the parts, timorousnesse, and an aptness to be frighted, with a sudden propensitie to fall into fits of the Mother, by reason of much bloud, oppressing and burthening the heart, also continuall anxiety, sadness, and want of sleep, with idle talking, and an alienation of the minde, but that which most commonly afflicts them, is a difficulty and paine to fetch their breath, for the chest by a continuall dialatation and compression, draweth the bloud from the *Matrix* to it selfe, in a large proportion, and sometimes produceth *asthmaticall* effects. But what shall we say concerning Widowes, who lye fallow, and live sequestred from these *Venereous* Conjunctions? we must conclude, that if they be young, of a black complexion, and hairie, and are likewise somewhat discoloured in their cheeks, that they have a spirit of salacity, and feel within themselves a frequent titillation, their seed being hot and prurient, doth irritate and inflate them to *Venery*, neither is this concupiscence allaid and qualified, but by provoking the ejaculation of the seed, as *Galen* propounds the advice in the example of a widow, who was afflected with intolerable symptomes, till the abundance of the spermatick humour was diminished by the hand of a skilfull Midwife, and a convenient oyntment, which passage will also furnish us with this argument, that the use of *Venery* is exceeding wholesome, if the woman will confine her selfe to the Lawes of moderation, so that she feele no wearisomnesse, nor weaknesse in her body, after those pleasing conflicts.[32]

There is a parallel, but much more concise, account by John Pechey (1655–1716), who unlike most of his contemporaries is familiar with the sexual function of the clitoris; he describes the "suffocation of the womb" as a disease caused by "the retention of the Seed" and cured by an "evacuation" of it either by intercourse or by the use of "odoriferous salves."[33]

The famous physician Thomas Sydenham (1624–89) believed that hysteria was responsible for about "one-sixth of all human maladies." In his "Epistolary Dissertation" he says:

> Of all chronic diseases hysteria—unless I err—is the commonest; since just as fevers—taken with their accompaniments—equal two thirds of the number of all chronic diseases taken together, so do hysterical complaints (or complaints so called) make one half of the remaining third. As to females, if we except those who lead a hard and hardy life, there is rarely one who is wholly free from them—and females, be it remembered, form one half of the adults of the world.[34]

If hysteria were merely the normal functioning of female sexuality, it would hardly be surprising that nearly all women showed symptoms, except perhaps those too exhausted by hard labor and short commons.

William Harvey, much better known for his work on the circulation of the blood than for his *Anatomical Exercitations concerning the Generation of Living Creatures* (1653), considered hysteria a terrible scourge among women, caused, in his view, by disorders of menstruation or by sexual deprivation:

> No man (who is but never so little versed in such matters) is ignorant, what grievous *symptomes*, the Rising, Bearing down and Perversion, and Convulsion of the *Wombe* do excite; what horrid extravagancies of minde, what Phrensies, Melancholy Distempers, and Outragiousness, the *preternatural Diseases* of the Womb do induce, as if the affected Persons were inchanted: as also how many difficult *Diseases*, the depraved effluxions of the Terms, or the use of *Venus*, much intermitted and long desired, do foment. [Emphasis in the original][35]

In "On Parturition" (1647) he had described the spasms or paroxysms of the female reproductive system during hysterical episodes and asserted that these occurred when "the passions are strong."[36]

Of all the seventeenth-century physicians who wrote on hysteria, the most matter-of-fact and morally unabashed was Nathaniel Highmore, whose *De Passione Hysterica et Affectione Hypochondriaca* of 1660 is one of the few medical works in Western history to straightforwardly

call the hysterical paroxysm an orgasm. He describes the engorgement of the female genitalia with blood during the arousal stage and the accompanying release of vaginal fluids. The paroxysm, he observes, constricts the blood vessels during the "crisis" and returns the blood to the central organs. Both his description and the word he uses—*orgasmum*, which has only one meaning in Latin—leave no doubt that he fully understands the sexual character of the release the patient experiences in the hysterical paroxysm.[37] He admits, however, that the technique of producing the desired crisis is difficult for physicians to learn. I shall return to this subject later. His account of the disease, however, was controversial in its time and virtually ignored in later centuries.[38]

The Eighteenth and Nineteenth Centuries

Hermann Boerhaave (1668–1738) refers to Aretaeus's description and treatment, recommending exercise, marriage, and massage for both female hysterics and male hypochondriacs.[39] In Boerhaave's day hypochondriasis did not mean a preoccupation with psychosomatic ailments but was the parallel to hysteria in women: a disorder of males caused by sexual deprivation. Not all physicians believed the disorder existed; Boerhaave, evidently, was one of the believers. Bernard Mandeville (1670–1733) seems to have thought that marrying off young women as a treatment for hysteria was old-fashioned, and in his *Treatise of the Hypochondriack and Hysteric Passions* of 1711 he prescribed horseback riding for hysterical young girls combined with a regimen of massage for up to three hours daily.[40] The same author, apparently deeply concerned about the insalubrious effects of sexual deprivation on humanity, published in 1724 a volume called *A Modest Defence of Publick Stews*. The anonymous author of the 1737 *Onania* differed from these views, asserting that hysteria, sterility, and leucorrhea were caused by masturbation. His recommended cure was traditional: marriage.[41]

Havelock Ellis, who surveys much of the literature of hysteria and sexuality in his *Studies in the Psychology of Sex*, mentions Albrecht von Haller (1708–77).[42] Ellis asserts that Haller "said that women are especially liable to suffer from privation of sexual intercourse to which they have become accustomed, and referred to chlorosis, hysteria, nymphomania and simple mania curable by intercourse." William Cullen (1710–90), a physician famous in his own and later times, wrote in his essay "On Hysteria or Hysteric Disease," in *First Lines of the Practice of Physic*, that it occurred "frequently in young widows. It occurs especially in those females who are liable to the Nymphomania; and the Nosologists have properly enough marked one of the varieties of the disease by the title of *Hysteria Libinosa*."[43] He refers to the engorgement of the blood vessels of the female genitalia during arousal, reminiscent of the plethora of pent-up fluids thought by his predecessors to require sexual purging, and likens it to the engorgement of blood vessels in the brain then thought to accompany epilepsy. Describing the hysterical paroxysm, Cullen notes that during it the entire abdominal area is contracted, including the anal sphincter, and that urination is entirely suppressed.

Joseph Raulin (1708–84) too, in his *Traité des affections vaporeuses du sexe* of 1758, mentions contractions or "local spasms" in hysterical fits. There are few if any human conditions other than orgasm that involve strong contractions of the vagina and anal sphincter. Certainly the characteristic orgasmic contractions of the uterus and vagina provide relief from the "symptoms" of arousal, and no doubt the patients of these physicians reported feeling much better for the experience.

Purportedly therapeutic experiences that sound remarkably similar to those described above were provided by less than reputable practitioners, such as Friedrich Anton Mesmer (1733–1815). Since he was not a physician, the social camouflage of medical practice did not extend to him, and thus he was widely suspected of stirring up sexual passions in his female patients. Similar doubts had been expressed about the ecstatic behavior of the female convulsionaries of Saint Médard, bishop of Vermandois (ca. 470–ca. 560) at the chapel of Abbé Paris.[44] Charles MacKay commented in 1841 on the predominance of women and girls among Mesmer's followers, describing a mesmeric session as follows: the women sat in a circle around a vessel of "magnetised water" and iron filings, holding hands and touching knees. "Assistant magnetisers, generally strong, handsome young men," came in and "embraced the patient between the knees," massaging her breasts and torso as they gazed into her eyes. "A few wild notes on the harmonica or piano-forte or the melodious voice of a hidden opera-singer" were the only sounds except, presumably, for the breathing of the magnetees. MacKay tells us that the women began to redden visibly, until "off they went, one after the other, in convulsive fits. Some of them sobbed and tore their hair, others laughed till the tears ran from their eyes, while others shrieked and screamed and yelled till they became insensible altogether." After the crisis, Mesmer himself entered and stroked the faces, spines, breasts, and abdomens of the "insensible," whereupon "they were restored to consciousness."[45]

One of the few medical writers in whose works the voice of a woman is heard on this subject, at least at second hand, is Franz Josef Gall (1758–1828), whom Havelock Ellis described as "a genius in isolation." A patient of his, a young widow, had been experiencing hysterical fits. Gall says that "the crisis never fails to terminate with a discharge that occurs with thrills of pleasure, and in a veritable ecstasy, after which she is free from attacks for a while."[46] At the same period, Philippe Pinel asserted that hysteria and nymphomania were caused by sexual frustration or masturbation, and that physicians should direct their efforts to bringing on the "évacuation sexuelle," as described by Gall.

It is at this point in our chronology, the beginning of the nineteenth century, that the nosological and etiological framework of hysteria becomes both confused and confusing. I warned earlier that the causal logic of my sources, if we may so dignify their reasoning, would become difficult to understand. The paradigm of hysteria as a disease, to use the terminology of Thomas Kuhn, had reached the point where it did not readily explain either the empirical data or the variations in them. The paradigm fragmented into three related disorders, of which one, chlorosis or "greensickness," had been known well before the nineteenth century, mainly to practitioners of what we now call "folk medicine."[47] The symptoms and etiologies of these three disorders overlapped substantially and were thought to be closely related. Ellis remarked in the early twentieth century that "as Luzet has said, hysteria and chlorosis are sisters." Physicians could not agree, however, whether sexual deprivation or overindulgence caused any of the disorders, and whether masturbation was a cause or a symptom of any of them. The debate was considerably muddled by the vague and poorly defined characters of all three ailments, a situation graphically illustrated in an anecdote from Jan Goldstein, who quotes "the psychiatrist Charles Lasègue, who pronounced hysteria 'the wastepaper basket of medicine where one throws otherwise unemployed symptoms.'"[48] I shall have more to say of this when I turn to the influence of Charcot and the Salpêtrière. Some physicians questioned the propriety of vulvular massage; Thomas Stretch Dowse in 1903 quoted the nineteenth-century author Douglas Graham, who said that "massage of the pelvic organs should be intrusted to those alone who have 'clean hands and a pure heart.'"[49]

Chlorosis or greensickness had a venerable tradition by this time as a disorder of young women, variously interpreted by modern historians as anemia, anorexia nervosa, or some combination of the two.[50] Folk traditions and some medical thought from the sixteenth century through the nineteenth attributed chlorosis to sexual deprivation in virgins—as Thomas Laycock put it in 1840, "excited love, [and] ungratified desire."[51] Mary Gove Nichols, of water cure fame, thought chlorosis was an effect of "solitary vice."[52] Its symptoms were protean, including everything from lassitude and nausea to sexual fantasy. Whatever the origins of the disease, its treatment was almost identical to treatments for hysteria, except that hydropathic physicians usually added iron to the patient's diet in the form of "chalybeate waters."

Neurasthenia was an invention of the second half of the nineteenth century, and those who believed in its existence considered it a new disease caused by the stresses of modern life. The diagnosis was popularized by George Beard, who published an influential work on neurasthenia in 1884.[53] As with hysteria and chlorosis, the interpretation of its supposed symptoms in women included many elements consistent with the normal functioning of female sexuality under social conditions that interpreted it as pathological. The plethora of possible etiologies was matched only by the bewildering array of symptoms. Haller says that "weeping, irritability, depression, mental and physical weariness, morbid fears, forgetfulness, palpitations of the heart, headaches, writing cramps, mental confusion, fear of impending insanity, and constant worry were the most noted symptoms." But almost anything could be a symptom of neurasthenia, including yawning, itching, stomach upsets, ticklishness, insomnia, and muscle spasms.[54] Daniel Brinton even went so far as to suggest that childbearing could cause neurasthenia, apparently making the Balboan discovery that caring for small children can cause sleeplessness and "mental and physical weariness."[55] By the end of the nineteenth century neurasthenia was frequently classed with hysteria and chlorosis under the generic term "hysteroneurasthenic disorders." Although marriage was rarely recommended as a treatment for neurasthenia, many of the other treatments were the same as those for hysteria and chlorosis, including massage. Neurasthenia was sometimes defined as "a slight hysterical tendency."[56] Men could also be neurasthenic; overwork, masturbation, and sexual excess were thought to be predetermining factors in males.[57] Ernest Jones asserted in 1918 that in neurasthenic women, "persistence of clitoris masturbation is one of the most important agents leading to (sexual) anaesthesia because it means fixation on the infantile, male form of sexuality."[58]

Throughout the nineteenth century, medical professionals struggled to bring scientific reasoning to the study of the hysteroneurasthenic disorders, with somewhat mixed success. R. J. Culverwell, for example, asserted in his 1844 *Porneiopathology* that although "continence in females" is thought "to be the brightest ornament a woman possesses," its effects are pathological, as "is truly attested by the miseries of hysteria, and other nervous derangements, that pervade the junior and elderly maiden branches of every family, and constitute so formidable an enemy to domestic felicity."[59] Robert Brudenell Carter, in *On the Pathology and Treatment of Hysteria* (1853), asserted that any repressed emotion could lead to hysteria, but the one most likely to cause trouble was sexual passion. Charles Delucena Meigs asked in the third (1854) edition of his widely read *Woman: Her Diseases and Remedies*, "What is her erotic state? what the Protean manifestations of that Life-force developed by a reproductive irritation which you call Hysteria?"[60] Something of a liberal on the question of hysteria in the mid-nineteenth century, Meigs believed that men could be hysterical as well, and that their attacks were accompanied by erections.[61]

James Manby Gully, a hydropathic physician whose love life later achieved a somewhat unwelcome notoriety, wrote in his heyday of the efficacy of hydriatic massage in hysteria and "nervous headache," which he considered curable by the douche therapy illustrated in chapter 1: "The douche is a very necessary part of the treatment; and, played well on the loins, tends powerfully to facilitate the uterine functions." Few women who have experienced water under pressure "played well on the loins" would be inclined to argue with him.[62] In 1909 Curran Pope wrote that "imperfect or unsatisfactory intercourse" could cause not only hysteria but amenorrhea (failure of the menses) and dysmenorrhea (painful menstruation). For these ailments, he recommended douche therapy to the "inner surface of the thighs." He stresses the point with his fellow physicians that they will have little difficulty persuading women to accept hydriatic massage, noting that "Douches are, as a rule, more agreeable to the majority of individuals than the other forms of hydriatic procedure . . . It sets the tissues in a vibration impossible to describe; experienced, it is never forgotten."[63]

The French physician Pierre Briquet (1796–1881) did not mince words about the sexual etiology of hysteria: he was quite certain it was caused by sexual frustration, including "les mauvais traitements" by husbands. Briquet claimed to have treated 430 hysterics by 1859, only the middle of his long career, and he asserted that a quarter of all women suffered from this disorder. He cites Galen and Forestus on the utility of "la titillation du clitoris" for producing the desired "évacuation" and describes the medical controversy surrounding this type of treatment. He goes on to remark that hysterics typically do not reach orgasm during intercourse and that "nymphomanie" or chronic arousal may be one of the sequelae.[64] Somewhat paradoxically, he claims that prostitutes, who do not, as he points out, reach sexual climax in intercourse with customers, become hysterical from masturbation, and that many consider early marriage a prophylaxis for hysteria.[65] Briquet is one of the few physicians who, like Highmore, seem to understand what is going on in both the diagnosis and the treatment of hysteria, and he is unabashed about his own therapeutic role. For this he was criticized by at least one of his colleagues, as we shall see.

Wilhelm Griesinger (1817–68), a well-known American physician of the second half of the nineteenth century, noted that "nymphomaniacal excitement" was a symptom of hysteria. He observed that many cases of hysteria were relieved by "local treatment" such as massage when all other therapeutic strategies failed. A true penetrationist of the old school, he thinks that hysteria cannot be caused by sexual frustration because of "its great frequency amongst married women—the frequent injurious influence of marriage, pregnancy and childbirth, and the frequency of the affection amongst prostitutes."[66] Briquet seems to have a much clearer understanding of the affliction in question; Griesinger cannot imagine that intercourse and penetration could fail to be satisfying.

Russell Thacher Trall, another American, who was associated mainly with the hydropathic school, wrote in 1873 that women, including but not of course limited to hysterics, were an economic godsend to the profession of medicine, claiming that "more than three fourths of all the practice of the profession are devoted to the treatment of diseases peculiar to women" and that of the annual estimated aggregate income of United States physicians of more than $200 million, "three-fourths of this sum—one hundred and fifty millions—our physicians must thank frail woman for."[67]

If the normal functioning of female sexuality was defined as a disease, women must have seemed frail indeed. During the decade in which Trall wrote these lines, the proceeds of treating women would have equaled just under half of the entire federal budget. In the nineteenth century, the supposed pathology of women's sexuality was extended to nearly every aspect of her physiology. Ann Wood, in a discussion of an 1855 work by Catherine Beecher, remarks on Beecher's apparent belief that women of her time were sick "because they were women. Most of the ailments that she records—pelvic disorders, sick headaches, general nervousness—were regarded as symptoms of 'female complaints,' nervous disorders thought to be linked with the malfunctioning of the feminine sexual organs."[68] Albert Hayes, writing of hysteria, chlorosis, and nymphomania in 1869, was one of many medical authors of his day who regarded the female reproductive tract as a veritable swamp, rife with pathogenic miasmas. "The strength of the reproductive force" in women, he argues, "irradiates every part of the frame . . . when disordered by whatsoever cause, it becomes capable of carrying confusion into every department, where it may rave and rage in its caprice and fury."[69]

C. Bigelow, writing in 1875, said, in a discussion of women patients dissatisfied with their marital sex lives, that "almost every physician of large practice has a circle of 'everlasting patients,' whom he visits and prescribes for once a week, on the average, for years." He considered that though husbands' overindulgence in intercourse was wearying to women, withdrawal (coitus interruptus) was the most frequent cause of hysteria, with its attendant congestion of the female genitalia. He cites the vaginal lubrication associated with hysteria as evidence for this hypothesis.[70] The French physician Auguste Tripier observed in 1883 that the convulsive crisis of hysteria "est de même quelquefois de la crise vénérienne" (is sometimes the same as the orgasm).[71] He had earlier identified some of these "quelquefois" as the therapeutic remedies applied by his colleague Pierre Briquet:

> Some among you will remember a treatment for hysteria everybody was talking about twenty-five or thirty years ago: I am talking about vulvular massage, recognized in ancient times and put back into practice by Briquet, who was ready to give it up after a brief trial; but he says nothing about it in his book except in connection with his predecessors and as a kind of historical footnote. Leaving aside paraphrases, I would like to point out to you that for a while Briquet was treating hysteria with masturbation, practiced more or less systematically by his interns. Now Briquet was a serious professional, a man of mature judgment, and it would not be right to take lightly a verdict which cannot fail either to make him a laughingstock or to put him in a difficult and absurd position . . .
>
> My own observations have led me to concede the usefulness, at least for a while, of the hysterical crisis, so I suggest that Briquet has replaced a spontaneous crisis with one that is clinically induced, similar if not identical, in order to achieve remission of the disease.[72]

Nineteenth-century physicians noted that their hysterical and neurasthenic women patients experienced traditional androcentric intercourse mainly as a disappointment. Richard von Krafft-Ebing, who thought that "woman . . . if physically and mentally normal, and properly educated, has but little sensual desire," nevertheless considered the failure of his female patients to enjoy sex a pathological condition. He notes both that neurasthenic and hysterical women thus fail in their duty to their husbands and also that sexual "anesthesia," again in the context of penetration, was widespread among supposedly normal women.[73] The French physician Jules Philippe Falret was completely unsympathetic to his female patients on these grounds, asserting that their failure to respond to marital intercourse predisposed them to seek immoral satisfaction elsewhere.[74] His colleague Gilles de la Tourette, whose book is illustrated with drawings of nude females in the throes of "hysterical convulsions," stresses the role of sexual disappointment in the etiology and symptomatology of hysteria: "The sexual act is for a hysteric nothing but a disappointment: she does not understand it; inspires in her an insurmountable repugnance." It is unclear from his account whether her lack of pleasure in marital sex is a cause or an effect of the supposed disease.[75] Like many others, he notes the characteristic "muqueuse vulvovaginale" of the active hysteric. These fascinations with fluids and with photography seem to have been fairly common in the French neurological community of the late nineteenth century. La Tourette's colleague at the Salpêtrière, Désiré Magloire Bourneville, had in 1878 published a massive three-volume medical work in which voyeuristic photographs of women stimulating their own nipples or arched in ecstatic paroxysms (with captions like "Lubricité") illustrate texts such as Bourneville's observations of "Th.," an eighteen-year-old diagnosed as hysterochlorotic. The physician notes with interest that she cries out "Oue! Oue!" tosses her head back and forth, and then rocks and flexes her torso very rapidly. "Then, her body curves into an arc and holds this position for several seconds. One then observes some slight movements of the pelvis." Shortly thereafter, "she raises herself, lies flat again, utters cries of pleasure, laughs, makes several lubricious movements and sinks down onto the vulva and right hip." The state of vaginal lubrication of these patients is noted at frequent intervals: "La vulve est humide" or "La sécretion vaginale est très abondante."[76] The vocalizations of these women and their *bavardage* (babble) during "les sensations volupteuses" were duly transcribed as well.

The American gynecologist William Goodell endorsed massage and electrotherapy in hysteria, "to promote the secretions" necessary to relieve the pelvic congestion that was, he said, one of the sequelae of unsatisfactory intercourse, particularly withdrawal. His patients reported a desire to sleep after treatment.[77] Another electrotherapist, Franklin Martin, noted that women are often exhausted from childbearing and from "excessive cohabitation," resulting in neurasthenia, one of the symptoms of which is that "the vagina is often sensitive, bathed with mucus frequently."[78] This preoccupation with lubrication appears also in the works of Friedrich Bilz, a European writer on natural healing, who noted that during hysterical attacks "the sexual parts secrete a slimy fluid." Bilz was of the opinion that sexual desire was increased, not decreased, in hysterical women, but that its expression was unwholesome, resulting in "self-abuse," a tendency toward erotic fantasies or "exciting literature," and seductive behavior toward males.[79] Pelvic massage and thigh affusions (of water) were recommended.

William Dieffenbach, a hydrotherapist of the turn of the century, wrote that the etiology of neurasthenia could include sexual excesses of any kind, whether of chastity or of indulgence, as well as unsatisfying marital sex: "Conjugal incompatibility, sexual excess, masturbation, sexual continence, habits of over-indulgence in coffee, tea, tobacco and alcoholic beverages."[80] In his opinion, vibratory and hydromassage treatments of the abdomen were indicated.

At the same period when Freud was publishing his new theories about the etiology of hysteria, others were struggling with the ancient problem of how the disease paradigm conformed (or did not) to prevailing hypotheses about sexuality. A.F.A. King, an obstetrician, set forth in the *American Journal of Obstetrics* in 1891 a theory that sexual hysteria in women was

> *not, strictly speaking, a disease at all,* but rather a mere modification in the physiological government of the body, executed by the automatic action of the ruling nervous system, *for some definite, natural purpose.* The ultimate objects that underlie all the functions of the body as they are determined by the government of the nervous system, are mainly two, viz., the *preservation of the life of the individual,* which comes first and is of first importance; and, second, the *preservation or perpetuation of the species.* From what we already know of hysteria, there is much to suggest that the hysteric process would be more nearly allied with the second object than with the first. [Emphasis in the original]

His thesis is that women fall into hysterical "fits" in order to attract the advances of men and to overcome their supposed natural reticence. In support of this, King makes twelve arguments, of which the following are notable:

> 4. Every woman who exhibits the phenomena of a hysteric attack is always *ashamed of it* afterwards—instinctively ashamed. She will always

deny, never acknowledge it; and when accused or told of it will become offended and angry. This is an inherited and fundamental feature of the process.

5. It occurs most often in single women, or rather in those, whether single or married, whose sexual wants remain ungratified."

He goes on to refer to the controversy over whether marriage is a suitable cure. He then adds, "The hysterical paroxysm is a *temporary and short affair*. The helpless creature, who seems to have lost all her senses and sensations, is in a few minutes up and about, apparently as well as ever." King postulates a situation in which some "aboriginal Venus" is found in a hysterical state by some "youthful Apollo of the woods," who then

> touches, moves and handles her at his pleasure; she makes no resistance. What will this primitive Apollo do next? He will cure the fit and bring the woman back to consciousness, satisfy her "*emotion*," and restore her "*volition*"—not by delicate touches that might be "agonizing" to her hyperesthetic skin, but by vigorous massage, passive motion, and succussion that would be painless. The emotional process, on the part of the woman, would end, perhaps, with mingled laughter, tears and *shame*; and when accused afterwards of the part which the ancestrally acquired properties of her nervous system had compelled her to act, as a preliminary to the event, what woman would not deny it and be angry? But the course of Nature having been followed, the natural purpose of the hysteric paroxysm accomplished, there would remain as a result of the treatment—instead of one pining, discontented woman—two happy people and the probable beginning of a third.[81]

In this male fantasy thinly disguised as medical speculation, hysteria is a natural process intended to promote coitus and pregnancy, even in the context of rape if necessary.

The Freudian Revolution and Its Aftermath

Sigmund Freud's clinical training in hysteria took place mainly at the Salpêtrière under the tutelage of the prevailing "master" of French neurology and psychiatry, Jean-Martin Charcot. Freud greatly admired and revered Charcot, and many of the teacher's ideas found their way into Freud's conceptual frameworks.[82] As I show in chapter 4, the Salpêtrière was an internationally famous center of experimentation with physical therapies for hysteria, including the use of vibratory mechanisms. In his later years Freud recounted a conversation between Charcot and P. Paul Brouardel that was to shape Freud's eventual theories of hysteria:

> At one of Charcot's evening receptions, I happened to be standing near the great teacher at a moment when he appeared to be telling Brouardel a very interesting story about something that had happened during his day's work. I hardly heard the beginning, but gradually my attention was seized by what he was talking of: a young married couple from a distant country in the East—the woman a severe sufferer, the man either impotent or exceedingly awkward. "Tâchez donc," I heard Charcot repeating, "je vous assure, vous y arriverez." Brouardel, who spoke less loudly, must have expressed his astonishment that symptoms like the wife's could have been produced by such circumstances. For Charcot suddenly broke out with great animation: "Mais, dans ces cas pareils c'est toujours la chose génitale, toujours . . . toujours . . . toujours"; and he crossed his arms over his stomach, hugging himself and jumping up and down in his own characteristic lively way. I know that for a moment I was almost paralysed with amazement and said to myself: "Well, but if he knows that, why does he never say so?" But the impression was soon forgotten; brain anatomy and the experimental induction of hysterical paralyses absorbed all my interest.[83]

Charcot's unwillingness to publish this hypothesis, and his admonition of "Tâchez donc" struck Michel Foucault as significant: "One must not speak of these 'genital causes': so went the phrase—muttered in a muted voice—which the most famous ears of our time overheard one day in 1886, from the mouth of Charcot."[84] There is certainly no mention of this concept in the *Clinical Lectures* of 1888.[85] Charcot's reticence about the sexual etiology of hysteria apparently fooled his biographer Georges Guillain, who denies that his subject ever considered any such hypothesis.[86]

In any case, the "most famous ears of our time" retained the information, and Freud was to rework it into a new conception of hysteria that completely altered the disease paradigm. In his *Autobiographical Study* he very nearly paraphrases Charcot's observation: "I do not think I am exaggerating when I assert that the great majority of severe neuroses in women have their origin in the marriage bed."[87] The editors of the Standard Edition of Freud's works note that Freud studied hysteria under Charcot before setting up his practice in Vienna in 1886, where "he relied on such currently recommended methods of treatment as hydrotherapy, electrotherapy, massage and the Weir-Mitchell rest-cure. But when these proved unsatisfactory his thoughts turned elsewhere."[88] One wonders whether it was the physician or the patient or both who found the results of Freud's experiments with physical therapies "unsatisfactory," but it hardly seems surprising that the man who, notoriously, did not know what women wanted was less than successful as a gynecological masseur.

Freud's article "The Aetiology of Hysteria" took the position that hysterics suffered not from sexual deprivation but from "lesions in consciousness" caused by childhood trauma. In the 1896 essay Freud assumes that the experiences of sexual molestation reported as childhood traumas were real; later he was to abandon this position and assert that it was the child's thoughts and fantasies of sexuality that caused the "lesions."[89] The hysterical disorder supposedly prevented the female patient from enjoying sex in the "normal" way, that is, in the form of heterosexual coitus. Fritz Wittels, in a strikingly misogynist account of Freud's theories on hysteria, said that "hosts of hysterical women reject sexuality in the form of coitus. Others manifest that hysterically heightened sex life which is, nevertheless, mere show and self-deception."[90] According to Havelock Ellis, Freud equated hysterical paroxysms with masturbation and thought them "an equivalent of coitus."[91] Clearly, the founder of modern psychoanalysis wanted to retain some of the sexual nuances of hysteria, including its traditional (but not exclusive) association with women, while at the same time propounding a new hypothesis about its origin. For Freud, as for his mentor Charcot, hysteria in both sexes was associated with contractures and functional paralysis.[92]

If hysteria had its origin in juvenile exposures to sexuality, whether real or imagined, the husbands and male lovers of adult women were entirely exculpated. They need not exert themselves to provide the cure in the marriage bed that Charcot had hinted at, since only a professional therapist like Freud could "talk out" the disease. This hypothesis proved so appealing that it soon eclipsed all other discourse about hysteria, neurasthenia, and chlorosis. Some mavericks like Wilhelm Reich continued to argue as late as 1927 that neurasthenia and hysterical neuroses in women were caused by lack of sexual gratification, but within a few decades Freud's became the dominant paradigm.[93] His definition was retroactively applied to all supposed cases of hysteria, modern or ancient, couched in terms that made it sound almost like a respectable medical diagnosis. Wesley says, "When the word hysteria is used alone, the reference is to *conversion hysteria*, a term coined by Freud. In this context, it means the appearance of an organic condition with no underlying organic causation."[94] Freud's view of hysteria redirected not only the attention of his colleagues in the psychological sciences but even that of historians making retrospective studies of the hysteroneurasthenic disorders.

The failure to make sense of hysteria after the Freudian revolution is epitomized in a 1953 article by George Swetlow, a professor of medicolegal jurisprudence at the Brooklyn Law School. Just after the end of hysteria's 2,500 years of acceptance as a disease paradigm, it is evident that neither Swetlow nor any other physician is quite sure what hysteria was. Swetlow says that it is "a strange disorder in that it takes a position midway between truth and deceit—not only may hysterical symptoms caricature almost any known disability due to actual tissue alteration, but at the same time it presents features hardly distinguishable from fraud." He goes on to attribute the Freudian etiology: "Forbidden wishes and longings totally unacceptable in a civilized society were never relinquished but merely postponed to a more propitious future."[95] In this model, it would be a marvel if any human being escaped the disease. Clearly, it was a paradigm that explained everything and therefore nothing.

Recent historiography has begun to address the gender issues implicit in the disease paradigm of hysteria. Since 1972 the subject has been taken up by a number of historians, among them Carroll Smith-Rosenberg, Barbara Ehrenreich, Michel Foucault, and Peter Gay. Smith-Rosenberg has postulated that hysteria in nineteenth-century women was a symptom or result of conflict between their hypersexualized role and the social denial of their overtly sexual feelings. This could be interpreted as an intellectually elevated argument for what I am proposing here in substantially more earthy terms. Whatever Smith-Rosenberg means by "conflict," she does not explicitly question the post-Freudian definition or symptomatology of hysteria and does not appear to see in the pre-Freudian disease paradigm the normal functioning of women's sexuality.[96] Barbara Ehrenreich and Deirdre English, in *Complaints and Disorders*, discuss the apparent "epidemic" of hysteria in the nineteenth century and describe it as a "new disease," without an examination of the antiquity of the disease paradigm or its fluid character over time. They do mention, however, that "female sexuality could only be pathological, so it was only natural for some doctors to test for it by stroking the breasts or the clitoris."[97]

Michel Foucault superficially addresses what he calls the "hysterization of women's bodies." His purpose, of course, is to describe broad social and medical trends, not to document details of how disease paradigms might have masked uncomfortable truths about women's sexuality:

> *A Hysterization of Women's Bodies:* a threefold process whereby the feminine body was analyzed—qualified and disqualified—as being thoroughly saturated with sexuality; whereby it was integrated into the sphere of medical practice, by reason of a pathology intrinsic to it; whereby, finally, it was placed in organic communication with the social body (whose regulated fecundity it was supposed to ensure), the family space (of which it had to be a substantial and functional element), and the life of children (which it produced and had to guarantee, by virtue of a biologico-moral responsibility lasting through the entire period of the children's education): the Mother, with her negative image of "nervous woman," constituted the most visible form of this hysterization.[98]

Without, again, addressing hysteria's long history before the nineteenth century, Foucault touches on a significant point: that women's sexuality was thought to require medical intervention. His discussion does not include the omission of female orgasm from the normative medical model of the nineteenth century, and he has little to say on what this might imply about hysteria. Like many others, he fails to question the disease paradigm itself: Why is this disorder so elastic in its boundaries that it can encompass such a broad spectrum of social goals?

Peter Gay, an unblushing fan of Sigmund Freud's contributions to human knowledge, erroneously attributes to him the invention of the idea that these "'noxae'—hysteria and anxiety neurosis" were caused by "a failure of sexual gratification, whether on the part of the man or the woman." Gay characterizes Freud's endorsement of a hypothesis at least as old as Hippocrates as "a radical departure."[99]

Freud's belief that men could be hysterical certainly was a minority opinion in his own and earlier times, but as we have seen, the concept of hysteria as a sequel of sexual deprivation had currency for many centuries before Freud's time. Oughourlian has a somewhat less sanguine view of Freud's achievement, pointing out that "we need only replace the word 'retention' in the theory of Galen . . . and in all those who were inspired by it during the next fifteen centuries or so with the term 'repression' . . . and replace 'purgation' with 'catharsis' to discover in all its supposed originality the Freudian theory of sexual neurosis."[100]

Although Gay's views on sexuality are, as we shall see, substantially androcentric, he does raise a question with real significance for understanding hysteria as a disease paradigm: "To deny women native erotic desires was to safeguard man's sexual adequacy. However he performed, it would be good enough. She would not—would she?—ask for more."[101] If she did, she could be labeled hysterical and sent to a doctor for treatment, thereby both removing the threat to her sexual partner's self-esteem and preserving the androcentric norm of penetration to male orgasm. It is to the persistent lure of this model of normal sexuality that we turn in the next chapter.

3

"My God, What Does She Want?"

Donald Symons, in his 1979 *Evolution of Human Sexuality*, says that female orgasm "inspires interest, debate, polemics, ideology, technical manuals, and scientific and popular literature solely because it is so often absent," unlike "the male orgasm, which exists with monotonous regularity and for the most part is interesting only to people directly involved in one."[1] As we observed in chapter 1, it has been clinically and popularly noted at many times and places that women do not reach orgasm during coitus as readily as men do, and that sustained stimulation of the clitoris is usually required to reliably produce the paroxysm described by Masters and Johnson as "a highly variable peak sexual experience accompanying involuntary, rhythmic contractions of the outer third of the vagina—and frequently of the uterus, rectal sphincter, and urethral sphincter as well—and the concomitant release of vasocongestion and muscular tension associated with intense sexual arousal."[2] This is, of course, a medical definition of orgasm: in this century as in previous ones, physicians are considered the experts on sexuality, and they carry much of the responsibility for establishing sexual norms.

In the second half of this century we have determined that most women do not have difficulty producing orgasm in themselves through masturbation, as Symons observes when he summarizes Kinsey's and Hite's research reporting that most women, like most men, can masturbate to orgasm in a little over four minutes, even though they rarely or never reach orgasm during intercourse. These authors "suggest that many women do not orgasm during intercourse, or do so sporadically, simply because sexual intercourse is an extremely inefficient way to stimulate the clitoris."[3]

Empirical studies have shown that women are not slower than men to become aroused and satisfied and that their orgasmic potential is much greater than that of males. In Kinsey's sample, 45 percent of the female masturbators reached orgasm in less than three minutes. Carol Tavris and Carole Wade pointed out in 1984 that "during masturbation, especially with an electric vibrator, some women can have as many as fifty consecutive orgasms," a figure that must have raised the ancient specter of female insatiability in more than one male mind.[4]

The lack of parallel experiences in intercourse for men and women flies in the face of both intuitive reasoning and cherished myth: How can it possibly be adaptive for women to experience orgasm primarily by some means other than the procreative act? How can it be that the act that socially and historically has defined masculinity and to which, to a significant extent, male sexual self-esteem is ultimately linked is not reliably rewarding to women? Why, indeed, do most women desire men at all, when intercourse so often proves a disappointment? Let me assert again that I will not be able to answer all these questions, especially those that relate to the mysteries of reproductive physiology. For example, why should the clitoris not be inside the vagina so as to receive stimulation more efficiently during penetration?[5]

What is really remarkable about Western history in this context is that the medical norm of penetration to male orgasm as the ultimate sexual thrill for both men and women has survived an indefinite number of individual and collective observations suggesting that for most women this pattern is simply not the case. Clearly there is a strong cultural motivation to deny the contrary evidence. Even when observers have made every effort to be objective and scientific, the androcentric bias has come through in the questions that are asked of the data and in the kind of data that are ruled out of bounds, as when Masters and Johnson selected their sample of married women to exclude all those who did not reach orgasm during intercourse.[6] The failure of traditional medical theory to understand the difference between male and female orgasmic experience has had far-reaching effects. All healthy women, according to the traditional medical view, desire penetration by males and are sexually incomplete and unsatisfied unless so penetrated. Thus a man who penetrates a women can think of himself as doing her a favor, contributing to her mental and physical well-being, especially if he makes her pregnant.[7] Women who desire or express sexuality outside this context have been perceived as flawed, sinful, or sick, and men consider themselves justified in imposing social and medical sanctions to get compliance with the normative model of female pleasure during heterosexual intercourse that reinforces male self-esteem.

Since women cannot alter their sexual physiology in order to achieve actual compliance (consistent orgasm during coitus), they have employed a variety of strategies to reconcile reality with the normative model. The intellectually convoluted character of some of these conceptual dodges, a few of which I shall enumerate below, is reminiscent of Ptolemy's ingenious and, for many centuries, persuasive efforts to explain the apparent motion of heavenly bodies without removing the earth from the center of the universe.[8] In both cases removing man (the gender is used advisedly) from the center of things would have required a thoroughgoing reevaluation of the entire framework of belief. To this day most men (and many women) resist reconceptualizing sexuality as something other than a hierarchy in which heterosexual coitus occupies the apex.

Physicians and the Female Orgasm

Since ancient times, physicians have employed five basic strategies to reconcile perceived female sexuality with androcentric norms. The first and least common, of course, was the "emperor's new clothes" approach: the straightforward acknowledgment that only a minority of women reach orgasm during penetration without clitoral stimulation. Opinions of this kind generally accompany recommendations that such stimulation be provided during or before coitus, not through masturbation. Second, some physicians (and historians, as we shall see) who wrote about female sexuality confused enjoyment and arousal with orgasm, conflating desire for heterosexual contact and "turgescence" of the female genitalia with orgasmic resolution. Third, as we have seen, the sexual symptoms called "hysterical paroxysm" were observed by doctors who seem to have had little or no experience with the kind of female orgasmic behavior described by Masters and Johnson. Fourth, many physicians of the nineteenth century combined this failure to recognize sexual behavior when they saw it with a conviction that most women lacked sexual feelings and desire. This last was true whether or not the physician in question believed frigidity and anorgasmia were healthy conditions; some felt that an absence of sexual feelings in women was a pathology caused by the stresses of modern life, corsetry, overindulgence in masturbation, or marital incompatibility. Finally, some medical authors omit all mention of female orgasm, even in discussing female sexuality.[9]

There are many historical examples of physicians' imposing conceptual frameworks on their clinical evidence that are difficult for modern observers to understand. It is important to recognize that it is not necessary to argue for conspiracy or even misogyny among doctors over time: the evidence suggests that physicians called disease paradigms as they saw them. Conceptual frameworks, as we have learned from many other historical contexts, can determine what observers actually see, and therefore what they report in their accounts of the observation. Thomas Laqueur cites significant examples of this in the evolution of concepts of male and female anatomy.[10] In an entirely different context, Mirko Grmek says that many ancient Greek physicians were simply defeated by the "two-sided causality . . . so complex that reason is no longer able to track down all the interconnections." It was easier to simply rule part of reality out of bounds than to try to make all the data fit the system.[11]

Ancient physicians as a rule had little to say on the subject of female orgasm, except to debate whether it was necessary for conception. Writings attributed to Aristotle, though probably not written by him, noted that women often have difficulty reaching orgasm in coitus. Äetius thought that "a certain tremor" indicated conception; Soranus believed that desire, not orgasm, was the important factor in pregnancy.[12] This debate continued until the twentieth century: Franz Josef Gall mentions it in his *Anatomie* (1810–19), and even authors of modern medical texts feel the need to assert that there is no known correlation between either desire and fertility or orgasm and conception.[13]

Medieval writers such as Avicenna and Giles of Rome thought that women experienced pleasure by receiving male semen. Although Avicenna, apparently a realist about female sexuality, was careful to caution his readers that this pleasure would not be adequate to satisfy the female partner, Giles and other writers preferred to think that nothing was required beyond male ejaculation. Danielle Jacquart and Claude Thomasset remark that "without casting doubt on the intentions of Giles of Rome, one might suggest that he supplied arguments capable of clearing the male of all responsibility in the woman's quest for pleasure."[14] Helen Lemay summarizes Avicenna's account of a woman's "three delights in intercourse: one from the motion of her own sperm, a second from the motion of the male sperm, and a third from the motion or rubbing that takes place in coitus." The physician cautions men that to be sexually satisfied the woman should experience her own "movements of the matrix" before the man ejaculates.[15]

In Tudor and Stuart England, prevailing medical beliefs were that orgasm was necessary for conception, that lack of sexual satisfaction, following Galen's teaching, caused unhealthful imbalances in the humors, and that orgasm provided an incentive for women to risk their lives in pregnancy.[16] Many works of this era discussed the role of the clitoris as the principal locus of sexual pleasure. Ambroise Paré expressed the view in 1634 that women with strong sexual desires, languid lifestyles, and hearty appetites were less likely than other women to suffer disorders of the menses, since their humors flowed more freely:

> There are some that are purged twice, and some thrice in a month, but it is altogether in those who have a great liver, large veines, and are filled and fed with many and greatly nourishing meats, which sit idely at home all day, which having slept all night doe notwithstanding lye in bed sleeping a great part of the day also, which live in a hot, moyst rainie and southerly ayre, which use warme bathes of sweet waters and gentle frictions, which use and are greatly delighted with carnall copulation: in these and such like women the courses flow more frequently and abundantly.[17]

Paré does not seem to entirely approve of these women, but their sexual enthusiasm forms part of his list of behaviors that promote a healthful flow of humors.

Women who wanted more sexual gratification than their partners were willing to provide, however, were serious threats to the androcentric and pro-natal model of sexuality: Abraham Zacuto wrote in 1637 that nymphomania "is a dreadful and odious ailment, for it interferes with intercourse and conception."[18] This concern persisted for centuries: Gall worried in 1825 about a patient of his, a prostitute who was not sexually satisfied by coitus, whom he diagnosed as an incurable nymphomaniac.[19] Nathaniel Highmore, writing in 1660, discussed orgasm in considerable detail, placing it in the context of the theory of humors. Blood rushed to the sexual organs during arousal, and it was unhealthful for it to remain there. Orgasm caused contractions that returned the blood to the rest of the body. The action of the lungs—the heavy breathing—assisted the process.[20]

William Cullen, a century later, was sure that "the exercise of venery certainly proves a stimulus to the vessels of the uterus; and therefore may be useful, when, with propriety, it can be employed." Like most of his contemporaries, he was concerned about the swollen condition of the female genitalia (it was not customary until the nineteenth century to distinguish the uterus from the vagina and external genitalia) and thought it must be pathological. He made analogies to the "distention of the vessels of the brain" in epilepsy and to the "turgescence of the blood in the vessels of the lung" in asthma, and he proposed that a similar "turgescence of blood in the uterus, or in other parts of the genital system, may occasion the spasmodic and convulsive motions which appear in hysteria."[21]

Relief from unhealthful congestion was, as we have seen, a standard refrain in medical discussions of the importance of orgasm to both men and women. Renaissance and later physicians who recognized the role of the clitoris in producing orgasm may have had reservations about stirring up women's passions by this means, but most of them agreed that unsatisfied sexual desire was unhealthful.

Views of female orgasm, although not of congestion, changed significantly between the mid-eighteenth century and the early nineteenth. In the nineteenth century the "orgasmic" (that is, turgescent or congestive) condition in women was supposedly relieved by the soothing effect of semen released into the vagina, in the manner suggested centuries earlier by Giles of Rome and others.[22] Thus, in this model ejaculation outside the vagina was conducive to "uterine disease," since the female genitalia did not receive the health benefits of male emission. Some physicians regarded all contraceptive practices as injurious to women for this reason.[23] The American physician C. Bigelow, writing in 1875, was one of many who subscribed to this view, asserting that withdrawal causes pelvic congestion and thus hysteria in women. He also warned against masturbation on the grounds that "many [women] experience the nervous orgasm or spasm, which acts as harmfully on them, when much indulged in, as on males." In intercourse, though, orgasm in women was considered healthful and medically desirable.[24]

William Goodell, a highly respected American gynecologist of the latter part of the nineteenth century, considered coitus interruptus unhealthful for women and recommended intercourse to male orgasm as a treatment for hysteria. He was highly articulate on the health benefits of ejaculate: "I believe that the semen itself, aided of course by the general relaxation following the crisis, has a special property of allaying the congestive orgasm and the vascular turgescence of venereal excitement." Notwithstanding the efficiency and convenience of this arrangement—at least to men—Goodell notes with concern the prevalence of pelvic congestion in women as a sequel to intercourse.[25]

The feminist and medical radical Edward Bliss Foote, who had been recently imprisoned for dispensing contraceptives, in 1901 took husbands to task for failing to understand their wives' sexual needs. He said that when the husband is brutish and insensitive, women are sexually unresponsive and that "with this state of apathy and aversion on the part of the female, intercourse is mechanical, and the contusions of her organs by the organ of the male, is just about as injurious as if a billet of wood were introduced instead of the organ which Nature intended." Like his colleagues, however, Foote considered coitus the norm for sexuality and did not approve of masturbation for either sex, on the grounds that it did not permit a healthy exchange of animal magnetism between the sexes.[26]

Others, such as the famous Richard von Krafft-Ebing, were unwilling to permit sexual pleasure to women even in the context of marital intercourse. He has often been quoted in the opinion that "woman, however, when physically and mentally normal and properly educated, has but little sensual desire. If it were otherwise, marriage and family life would be empty words." Clearly he regards women's sexuality as a significant threat to social stability. The androcentric picture is completed by his flat assertion that "the distinctive event in coitus is ejaculation." He opposed masturbation in both sexes, claiming that it weakened desire for the opposite sex.[27]

Other doctors observed that women "learned frigidity" by a lack of satisfaction in marriage: where disappointment was the rule, women simply ceased to take any interest in the proceedings.[28] G. Kolischer wrote in 1905 in the *American Journal of Obstetrics:*

> Sexual excitement, not brought to its natural climax, the reaction leaves the women in a very disagreeable condition, and repeated occurrences of this kind may even lead to general nervous disturbances. Some of these unfortunate women learn to suppress their sexual sensation so as to avoid all these disagreeable sequelae. Such a state of affairs is not only unfortunate, because it deprives the female partner of her natural rights, but it is also to be deplored because it practically brings down such a married woman to the level of the prostitute.[29]

The French physician Gilles de la Tourette saw this process as part of the cycle of hysteria: the "frigid" hysteric is disappointed by coitus and communicates her distaste to her husband. His resentment and rejection then contribute to the development of her pathology.[30]

Even doctors who understood the function of the clitoris did not want to give up the comforting notion of female orgasm in coitus. Theodore Thomas, for example, wrote in 1891 that the purpose of the clitoris was "to furnish to the female the nervous erethrism which is necessary to a perfect performance and completion of the sexual act" and went on to observe that orgasm could be produced by clitoral stimulation "outside of intercourse."[31] Many physicians warned against manipulation of the clitoris, either by husbands or by the women themselves. Smith Baker said in 1892 that a common "source of marital aversion seems to lie in the fact that substitution of mechanical and iniquitous excitations affords more thorough satisfaction than the mutual legitimate ones do."[32] Thus

one of the perceived health risks of unsatisfactory coitus for women was that it could lead to masturbation.

Masturbation

Physicians until the second half of this century have traditionally been deeply suspicious of the pleasure women had in masturbation, and not only for the reasons they condemned or questioned it for males. Havelock Ellis, who wrote synopses of what most of his illustrious predecessors had to say about female sexuality, thought that after adolescence "masturbation is more common in women than in men." He thought it likely that all widows and single divorced women masturbated, which concerned him because he concurred with his colleague Smith Baker, who believed that masturbation caused "marital aversion" in women. He says of this that healthy and vigorous "women living a life of sexual abstinence, have asserted emphatically that only by sexually exciting themselves, at intervals, could they escape from a condition of nervous oppression and sexual obsession which they felt to be a state of hysteria." This view, of course, was not far removed from the earlier perspective on hysteria as the sequel of sexual deprivation. The most disquieting female masturbators, from the physicians' point of view, were the married women, whose behavior raised doubts about the ideal of mutual bliss in coitus. Like others of Ellis's contemporaries, some of whom I have quoted, Alfred Adler was convinced that married women masturbated because coitus so often failed to satisfy them.[33] It is likely that this observation was the source of many physicians' discomfort with the notion of female masturbation: it conflicted at a literally visceral level with the androcentric paradigm.

Despite its obvious efficacy in relieving pelvic congestion, in the eighteenth and nineteenth centuries the "mechanical and iniquitous excitations" of masturbation were thought to cause all manner of diseases and disorders in both sexes. Doctors thought they saw serious somatic symptoms of the practice: sunken eyes with black bags under them, pallor, general weakness, and a host of sexual manifestations that one physician, N. Cooke, described as necessarily culminating, eventually, in a massive, spasmodic system failure, a sort of death by orgasm. Of female masturbation Cooke exclaims, "Alas, that such an expression is possible!" and goes on to cite the practice as the chief cause of nymphomania.[34] Sewing machines, particularly the kind with two foot treadles operated alternately, were thought by many nineteenth-century physicians to be either the cause or the means of masturbation in women, a concern also expressed about the bicycle.[35] According to Krafft-Ebing, the French writer A. Coffignon thought that the power of the sewing machine was such that heterosexual women could be turned into lesbians by "excessive work" on them.[36] Thomas Low Nichols considered masturbation a major source of pregnancy complications.[37]

E. H. Smith, in the *Pacific Medical Journal* of 1903, was so concerned about the possibility of his colleagues' failing to diagnose masturbatory diseases in their female patients that he published a guide to detecting masturbation by examination. A woman with one labium longer than the other, he asserted, had caused this "hypertrophy" by masturbating on that side. Since the relative sizes of the labia, like those of hands, feet, ears, and testicles, are usually determined by laterality, Smith must have discovered multitudes of female masturbators by this method. Passing a "mild faradic current" through the urethra was another method of determining whether women were more sexually sensitive than Smith thought was good for them.[38]

Nearly all female disorders could be attributed to masturbation or related sins, such as drinking alcohol, tea, or coffee, thinking about sex, or "tight corsets worn while reading French novels."[39] Mary Gove Nichols, a hydropathic physician, Grahamite, and "sexual radical," thought that menorrhagia and dysmenorrhea could be caused either by masturbation or by "excessive indulgence of amativeness" with one's spouse.[40] Russell Thacher Trall, another water cure physician, concurred with both views.[41] Trall thought intercourse was especially dangerous for women who constricted their organs with tight corsetry.[42] These conservative views on coitus may have increased the popularity of hydropathic physicians with women, who represented the major market for their services.

George Beard, whom I have mentioned as the great popularizer of neurasthenia, believed that masturbation "is almost universal. It is indulged in by both sexes." But excessive indulgence could have pathological sequelae in some persons of weak constitution: "It is the masturbation acting on a nervous diathesis, it is the habit *plus* a nervous constitution that gives us the product—sexual neurasthenia."[43]

Even while condemning female masturbation, some physicians were apparently comforted by the unsupported assumption that most women accomplished this forbidden act by some means approximating coitus. As early as the thirteenth century, Arnaldus of Villanova had recommended the use of a dildo to widows and nuns suffering from the dread symptoms of hysteria.[44] Any object or device that traveled the path of the totemic penis into the vagina was, at the end of the nineteenth century, suspected of having an orgasmically stimulating effect. The widespread adoption of the speculum as a medical instrument was far more controversial than that of the vibrator a few years later.[45] Elaborate tales were related of women and girls lusting after medical examination and climaxing on the examining table the minute the speculum was inserted. Robert Carter, a British physician and social critic, wrote of the speculum in 1853:

> No one who has realized the amount of moral evil wrought in girls . . . whose prurient desires have been increased by Indian hemp [marijuana] and partially gratified by medical manipulations, can deny that remedy is worse than the disease [hysteria]. I have . . . seen young unmarried women, of the middle-class of society, reduced by the constant use of the speculum to the mental and moral condition of prostitutes; seeking to give themselves the same indulgence by the practice of solitary vice; and asking every medical practitioner . . . to institute an examination of the sexual organs.[46]

To modern women, for whom pelvic examinations are a routine ordeal (and perhaps for Carter's female contemporaries), these assertions seem strange indeed. Opponents of the speculum also argued that its use required looking at the patient's genitalia, a clearly indelicate situation. The earlier method of examination, called "the touch," did not even require the patient to disrobe completely.[47] Part of the attraction of the new technology, however, was that the physician could greatly reduce tactile contact with the patient. One of the inventors of the speculum, gynecologist James Marion Sims, asserted that a significant component of his motivation for experimenting with the new technology was simple distaste: "If there was anything I hated," he wrote in 1884, "it was investigating the organs of the female pelvis."[48] In any event, the medical profession adopted the speculum, apparently deciding that its advantages as a diagnostic tool outweighed its perceived (and probably imaginary) dangers as a masturbatory device. The belief that most women masturbated with penis substitutes (dildos) must have been very comforting, but only about 11 to 20 percent of modern women surveyed actually use such methods.[49] In 1980 it was estimated that some form of masturbation was practiced by 97 percent of males and 78 percent of females; we do not, of course, have acceptable estimates for previous centuries.[50]

At the end of the nineteenth century the masturbation issue was open to considerable debate. Freud began to doubt in 1896 that masturbation caused neuroses, although he was still willing to believe it caused bed-wetting, leucorrhea, and some kinds of hysteria.[51] Robert Taylor, writing in 1905, warned that horseback riding, use of sewing machines, and bicycle riding could all lead to female masturbation, but that "in general no great harm is done to the system by the habit." An exception was vaginismus, which he thought could be caused by masturbating with a dildo or similar object. He attributes the prevalence of female masturbation among married women to the potential frustrations of intercourse: "In many cases the too rapid completion of the sexual act in the man leaves the woman unsatisfied, and she as a result produces the orgasm upon herself at the first opportunity."[52]

"Frigidity" and Anorgasmia

It is in the nineteenth century that we see the fullest flowering of the third and fourth approaches to reconciling perceptions of women's sexuality with their observed behavior: believing either that women enjoyed intercourse sufficiently with or without the resolution now medically defined as orgasm, or that normal women experienced no sexual feelings at all. Both views assisted in the camouflage of orgasmic treatments, since in the first case no penetration (and therefore nothing sexual) was occurring during the treatment and in the second case sexual pleasure on the

part of the patient was theoretically impossible. Belief in female frigidity or in women's total indifference to sexual stimuli was popular with both physicians and the public. One theory was that in the hysteric, frigidity and insatiability were combined in women who went from lover to lover seeking the gratification that a supposedly normal female would have experienced in coitus with her spouse. Madame Bovary was regarded as the epitome of this type, but the stereotypically insatiable female was hardly a newcomer (so to speak) to literature.[53] Nineteen centuries before Flaubert, Juvenal, who aimed his longest satire at the opposite sex, had expressed the characteristic male fear and disgust at the ability of women to have intercourse repeatedly without reaching orgasm, and their ability to achieve orgasm with external stimulation alone. Writing ostensibly to dissuade a young friend from marrying, Juvenal described "an imperial whore" who goes out for a long and active night of paid sex, after which "she sadly departed/Last of them all to leave, still hot, with a woman's erection,/Tired by her men, but unsatisfied still, her cheeks all discolored." Later in the poem the imaginary wife of his friend is at the bathhouse, where massage is apparently the chief attraction: "then it is time for the man with the oil to give her rubdown. Don't think that's all he does—his fingers are certainly clever,/Knowing where they can go, and how they can work up a climax."[54] A decorous and loyal frigidity in one's wife, in this model, seems to have been regarded as preferable to a passionate temperament beyond the husband's power to satiate it.[55]

Physicians, popular culture, and even some feminists attempted in the nineteenth century to establish decorous anorgasmia as a normal, even desirable, feminine trait. In 1844 the French physician Adam Raciborski had asserted that "three-fourths of women merely endure the approaches of men."[56] Carl Degler reports that Charles Taylor wrote in 1882 that "women have 'less sexual feeling than men' and that some people even go so far as to claim that 'as a rule women have practically nothing of what is understood as sexual passion.' As many as three-quarters of married women, he had been told, took no pleasure in the sexual act."[57] The ideal of passionlessness appealed to many women of Taylor's time, for whom intercourse without orgasm but with the danger of pregnancy and all its potential pains, complications, risks, and costs in time and health must have been a much less attractive prospect than to their relatively unencumbered male partners. William Hammond wrote in

1887 that "leaving prostitutes out of consideration, it is doubtful if in one-tenth of the instances of intercourse [women] experience the slightest pleasurable sensation from first to last."[58] Hermann Fehling asserted in 1893 that "it is an altogether false idea that a young woman has just as strong an impulse to the opposite sex as a young man . . . The appearance of the sexual side in the love of a young girl is pathological." He goes on to say that "half of all women are not sexually excitable."[59] Havelock Ellis commented in 1910 that "by many, sexual anesthesia is considered natural in women, some even declaring that any other opinion would be degrading to women; even by those who do not hold to this opinion it is believed that there is an unnatural prevalence of sexual frigidity among civilized women."[60] In his "Sexual Impulse in Women," he cites a number of medical authors who claim "frigidity" rates of between 66 and 75 percent for "civilized women," numbers that are suggestively similar to Shere Hite's late 1970s figures for women who do not regularly reach orgasm in coitus.[61] Sophie Lazarsfeld in the mid-twentieth century said that "the proportion of frigid women, according to the scientific investigators, varies between 60 and 90 per cent."[62] Of this reportedly rampant female frigidity in the late nineteenth and early twentieth centuries, John D'Emilio and Estelle Freedman point out that this view had attractions for some women, since it suggested "spiritual equality" with man and implied that "purity could be a useful tool with which women could gain leverage in sexual relations, for it provided them with grounds for refusing unwanted sex."[63]

There must have been a good deal of this last, because the same authors comment on the results of Clelia Mosher's survey of 1900–1920 that "half of these women expressed sexual desires and found sex agreeable, at least 'at times,' but more telling was the fact that even those who felt no desire participated in regular sexual relations." D'Emilio and Freedman go on to say that "most [nineteenth-century] women who complained that their husbands neglected marital sexuality stressed their desire for children rather than their desire for physical pleasure."[64] The American physician Elizabeth Blackwell subscribed to this view.[65] If only a minority of women had regular orgasmic experience in coitus, the majority's lack of interest is understandable: Why bother?

Laqueur says of Freud that "in 1905, for the first time a doctor claimed that there were two kinds of [female] orgasm and that the vaginal sort was the expected norm among adult women."[66] Freud was certainly the great popularizer of this androcentric theory, but he was not the first to raise the question of where the female orgasm originated. The subject was clearly a matter for debate when Auguste Tripier asserted in 1883 that clitoral and uterine sensations had to occur simultaneously for the production of the "venereal orgasm in women."[67]

It was twentieth-century post-Freudian medicine, however, that elevated the vaginal orgasm to a veritable Holy Grail of sexual function for women. When Alfred Kinsey dared to question both its existence and the necessity for adjusting women's sexuality to fit an inappropriate "norm," some of his colleagues reacted with horror and outrage. Edmund Bergler and William S. Kroger, who defined frigidity as "the incapacity of woman to have *a vaginal orgasm during intercourse*" (italics in the original), responded to Kinsey's book on female sexuality with eloquent indignation:

> The frigid women (not a mere 10 per cent as Kinsey assumes from the application of his mistaken yardstick [i.e., whether women could reach orgasm by any means], but probably 80 to 90 per cent) received the assurance that vaginal frigidity is a meaningless concept, and that the "normal" expectation is some form of clitoridean orgasm. This can be proved by an admission made by Kinsey on page 584 of Volume II. In his heated polemic against the existence of vaginal orgasm, he claims that "*some hundreds* of the women in our own study have consequently been much disturbed by their failure to accomplish this biological impossibility." Obviously, Kinsey reassured these neurotics.[68]

Bergler and Kroger insist that there is no scientific difficulty with arguing that 80 to 90 percent of all women are "abnormal" and go on to defend the Freudian notion that real women are satisfied only by penetration. To give these authors their due, they are at least evenhanded about their normative illusions: they assert that "mature, normal men do not desire sex except with women they love tenderly."[69]

Having reaffirmed the norm as coitus, twentieth-century physicians tended to blur the distinction between orgasm and satisfaction much as their nineteenth-century predecessors had done. A propensity to equate enjoyment of coitus with orgasmic satisfaction remains embedded in both medical and popular discussions despite nearly a century of study of female sexuality. Women themselves do not always know how to answer questions that distinguish between pleasure and orgasm, just as men typically, in Paul Gebhard's words, "do not understand inquiries about differences between orgasm and satisfaction."[70] For most men, apparently, orgasm *is* satisfaction. Women, however, traditionally have been expected to find enjoyment in an activity—coitus—that results in orgasm for women in only a minority of instances. Thus women's pleasure in sex, which may consist of arousal, enjoyment of physical intimacy, or the expression of affection it represents for both partners, is routinely interpreted both by scientists and even by some historians as orgasmic experience, whether or not it actually is. Both Katherine Bement Davis's 1,183 college-educated respondents and James Cooper's later working-class and lower-middle-class sample, surveys reported in 1925 by Robert Dickinson and Henry Pierson,[71] were frequently uncertain what was meant by the term "orgasm." As we have seen, their doctors were not always certain either. Among women reporting sexual pleasure, including "orgasm" however defined, it has been observed that "peaks of feeling" short of clinically defined climax are frequently reported as orgasm.

Jeanne Warner, who wrote about this in 1984, used Joseph Bohlen's 1981 definition: "Only the unique waveforms of anal and vaginal pressure associated with the reflexive contractions of the pelvic muscles provide distinct physiological evidence of orgasm." In the absence of these signs, the emotional and physical enjoyment that women experience in coitus is frequently elevated to the stature of orgasm, both in the women's own reports and in their medical interpretation. Women are under pressure to appear normal and feminine in their sexual responses—defined, of course, in terms of the androcentric model—and physicians have traditionally sought evidence that validated this model. Warner thinks it likely that female orgasm in coitus is substantially overreported owing to women's tendency to say what their husbands and doctors want to hear, and she adds:

> Another factor in the denial of lack of female orgasm has to do with a male bias for phallic stimulation. Although hard data on the relationship between mode of stimulation and female response are lacking at present, the literature conveys a strong impression that the penis is not the most effective means of producing a maximal level of arousal and response for a woman. Those male authorities who advocate the superiority of emotional orgasm in women ["peaks of feeling"] suggest that whatever provides the greatest satisfaction for the male should also provide the greatest pleasure for the female. It is not easy for any woman, professional or otherwise, to suggest that the culturally ingrained symbol of "manhood" is not the ultimate sensual magic wand.[72]

In Dianne Grosskopf's sample of 1,207 women, commissioned by *Playgirl* and published in 1983, "masturbation was shown to be the most reliably orgasmic sexual practice." Grosskopf, like Warner, thought her respondents overreported orgasm with penetration, and she observed that "women appeared to be defensive and sometimes less than honest in their answers to the questions about orgasms." Significantly, she also reports that "all but a small number (20 percent) of respondents said they did not feel cheated if they did not experience orgasm during sex," and that "three-quarters of the women felt it more important for their partner to be pleased than for themselves to be pleased."[73] Gebhard, too, said that 57 percent of his sample reported themselves as "satisfied" without orgasm.[74] Clearly these women saw no reason to expect orgasmic satisfaction in coitus, felt uncomfortable with questions that would reveal their lack of conformity to the androcentric norm in this regard, and were motivated to stress the satisfaction of delivering acceptable sexual services to their male partners. In 1985 Ann Landers's newspaper column shocked the masculine world by reporting the results of her inquiries to readers about how they felt about "the act": of more than 100,000 women who responded, 72 percent wrote to say they'd much rather be doing something else.[75] It has been argued that these and other data, notably Hite's, contain a self-selection bias. This is certainly true, but it is difficult to imagine how we might gather data on human sexuality without introducing self-selection bias, observer effects, or other distortions.

Like that of physicians and other male professionals, the work of some male historians suggests they are anxious to interpret the highly ambiguous evidence on female sexuality in such a way as to reinforce the androcentric model. Peter Gay, in filling volumes with extrapolations from somewhat scanty data, has not hesitated to assume that all female assertions of pleasure in heterosexual activity indicate regular experience of orgasm. In a section of *The Education of the Senses* appropriately titled "The Dubious Certainty of Numbers," he consistently assumes female orgasm during penetration and conflates pleasure with orgasmic satisfaction, despite the clearly emotional, rather than physiological, tone of most of his quotations from women. Although he says that doctors' reports "testify to a brimming reservoir of unsatisfied female desire," Gay never questions that a woman's claim to enjoy sex means orgasm in coitus, even when his sources explicitly deny any sensual dimension to their pleasure.[76]

Carl Degler's work on female sexuality exhibits the same androcentric bias as Gay's. In his famous article "What Ought to Be and What Was," he addresses questions raised by the Mosher survey at the turn of the century. On his own evidence, neither women nor their physicians could distinguish among arousal, the "psychic and subjective" enjoyment of sex, Warner's "peaks of feeling," and the physiological orgasm as defined above. Without inquiring what Mosher's respondents might have meant by "venereal orgasm," as we have seen, a more ambiguous term when applied to women than when applied to men, Degler concludes from his evidence that 95 percent of Mosher's sample of forty-five women experienced orgasm in coitus. Degler's point is that what physicians asserted about female sexuality and what women experienced were probably very different, a point certainly worth making. Unfortunately, his use of the Mosher data is tendentious and misleading; later in the same article he misinterprets Kinsey's data in a manner that would have horrified Kinsey.[77] Like traditional physicians and many others of his historical and contemporary brethren, Degler is reluctant to rock the boat of the androcentric model of female sexuality. Katherine Nelson, in a passage quoted in Marie Stopes's *Married Love*, shows a different view of women's experience of sex in the early decades of this century:

To mate with men who have no soul above
Earth grubbing; who, the bridal night, forsooth,
Killed sparks that rise from instinct fires of life,
And left us frozen things, alone to fashion
Our souls to dust, masked with the name of wife—
Long years of youth—love years—the years of passion
Yawning before us. So, shamming to the end,
All shrivelled by the side of him we wed,
Hoping that peace may riper years attend,
Mere odalisques are we—well housed, well fed.[78]

The overloaded and leaking vessel of androcentric sexuality, as we have seen, has required systematic bailing out of contradictory data. Some of this has been accomplished, I have suggested, by medicalizing the production of female orgasm, thus relieving husbands and lovers of the chore of stimulating the clitoris, a task rarely compatible with such reliable masculine favorites as coitus in the female-supine position. Physicians did not relish the job either, however lucrative it might be as an office visit cash cow, and from ancient times to the end of the nineteenth century they sought some means of literally getting the female orgasm off their hands. Their efforts to mechanize and expedite the task while retaining the profitable character of orgasmic treatment are the subject of the next chapter.

4

"Inviting the Juices Downward"

In a discussion of electromedical technologies new in his day, in 1903 Samuel Howard Monell effectively summarized the demand of physicians since Hippocrates for some simple means of getting results with their hysterical patients: "Pelvic massage (in gynecology) has its brilliant advocates and they report wonderful results, but when practitioners must supply the skilled technic with their own fingers the method has no value to the majority." For physicians in this line of work, the vibrator was a godsend: "Special applicators (motor driven) give practical value and office convenience to what otherwise is impractical."[1]

Not only the need for skill but the time required annoyed physicians. Samuel Spencer Wallian, extolling the virtues of "rhythmotherapy" with a vibrator in 1906, asserted that in manual massage the physician "consumes a painstaking hour to accomplish much less profound results than are easily effected by the other [the vibrator] in a short five or ten minutes."[2] For the profitability of a physician's practice, at any period in history, the difference between ten minutes and an hour to complete treatment would have been significant.

As I mentioned earlier, at no time did physicians show any real enthusiasm for treating hysteria in their women patients. All the evidence points to their having generally considered it a tedious, difficult, and time-consuming chore and having made efforts to delegate the task to subordinates or machines even in ancient and medieval times. Western physicians have in general found physical therapies annoyingly labor intensive, an attitude that eventually resulted in an occupational split between doctors and physical therapists in the twentieth century. There had been earlier efforts in this direction, as we have seen; massage was often a lower-status task relegated to semiprofessionals at ancient and medieval bathhouses and at spas in the modern period. Until the nineteenth century, pelvic massage of women, useful in childbirth as well as in the treatment of hysteria, was not uncommonly the responsibility of midwives, whether or not under the supervision of a physician. As a mode of therapy, massage rarely was harmful, often was beneficial, and achieved results, if any, only with patience, which meant that from the Galenic physician's point of view it lacked the heroic character of surgery, venesection, and purging. In this context it is hardly surprising that physicians sought technologies that would allow them to reap the economic benefits of pelvic massage, as delegating it to another therapist did not, while avoiding a wearying and costly investment of the doctor's time and skill.

One of the first technologies used for this purpose was a retrofit of the water-powered saw. Although there is no evidence these devices were ever applied to gynecological treatment, some writers assert that in ancient times the vibrating beam ends of water-powered saws were sometimes padded with fabric and used for massage.[3] More often, those seeking physical therapies in ancient and medieval times employed manual massage providers, as did Juvenal's subject, or visited baths with appliances for pumping water under at least some pressure, even if only that of gravity. In 1734 one Abbé St. Pierre is reported to have invented a mechanical predecessor to the vibrator called a *trémoussoir*, but little is known about the use and configuration of this device.[4] Bathing and hygiene establishments offered simple adjuncts to manual massage at least as early as the Renaissance and possibly before (fig. 8), including hand-held beaters, kneaders, and brush-type stimulators of the kind now associated with saunas.

At the same time, there existed a set of technologies for treating vaginal and uterine disorders that necessarily overlapped with massage, since hysteria and chlorosis were both thought to be uterine in origin.

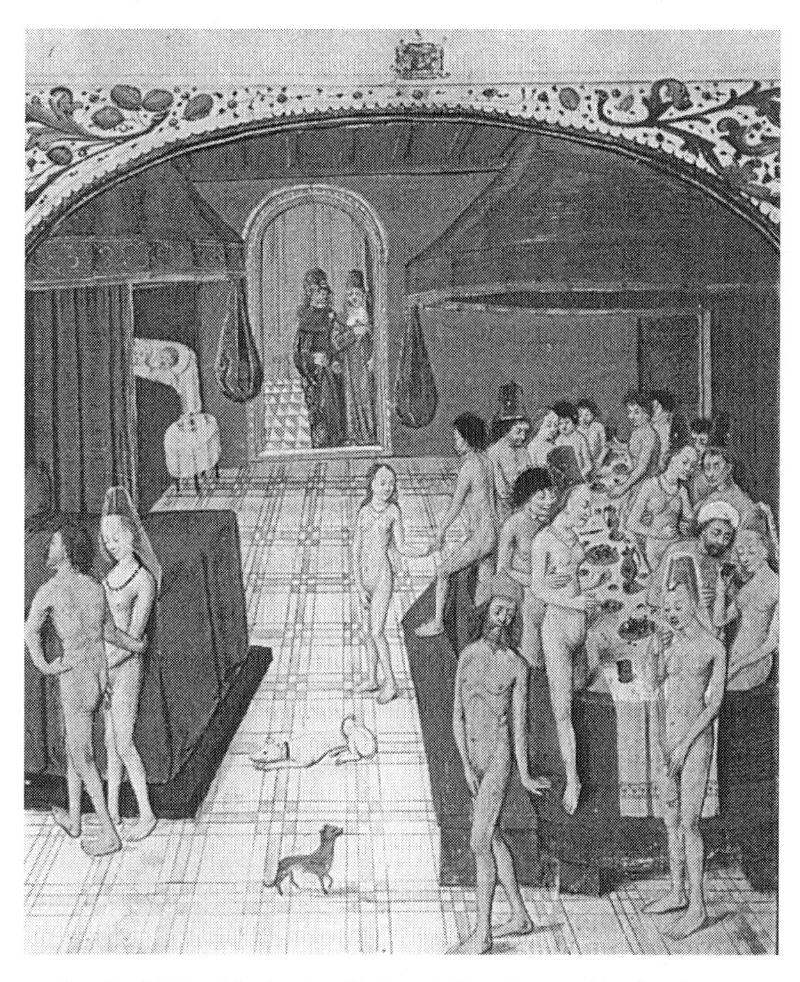

FIG. 8. Medieval bathing establishment. From Emmett Murphy, *Great Bordellos of the World* (1983), Bibliothèque Nationale.

Pessaries or suppositories containing Galenically cooling or heating ingredients, depending on the malady, could be prescribed. Another technique was subfumigation, illustrated in Paré, in which the patient sat over a small burner from which attractive or repellent fumes, again depending on the ailment, wafted upward into the vagina.[5] The efficacy of this method was thought to be enhanced by the use of perforated pessaries that held the vagina open to permit passage of the odoriferous vapors (fig. 9).[6]

As I indicated in chapter 2, massage of the vulva was a somewhat controversial practice among physicians after the medieval period, despite the treatment's venerable history. In the nineteenth century, the conflict and ferment of ideas about women and their physicians brought these debates into unaccustomed prominence. Public awareness of controversies among physicians had been growing steadily, of course, since the late Renaissance, when medical works began to abandon the international standard of Latin as the language of professional communication.[7] The trend was accelerated by the spread of inexpensive printing methods and materials that brought books within the economic reach of a much broader range of social classes in the nineteenth century. By 1890 the European or American lay reader of medical works had almost as many opportunities for exposure to medical confusion, controversy, and tendentious case studies as do modern viewers of television health programs. Although doctors had always attacked each other's theories and practice in their professional literature, the print explosion of the nineteenth century set the debate over clinical issues before the reading public for the first time. Physicians with radical ideas about therapy, such as the hydropaths who abounded in nineteenth-century America, Britain, and Europe, were especially likely to take their case to the customer rather than to their medical colleagues, who regarded their claims as questionable at best.

The direct massage of the vulva in hysteria and related disorders remained substantially unchanged through the nineteenth century. There was, however, a difference in the way the subject was discussed in some of the medical literature, particularly in America and Britain. Physicians were less likely than their predecessors, who could draw the veil of Latin over their expositions, to dwell on the details of their manipulations of the female genitalia, knowing that texts in the vernacular might well fall into the hands of the medically unqualified. Theodore Gaillaird Thomas mentioned gynecological massage treatments in a medical work published in Philadelphia in 1891, omitting any practical instructions on the grounds that "the details of the manipulations are too minute for reproduction here, and must be read in the original works," some of which were in Latin.[8] The French author A. Sigismond Weber, however, showed

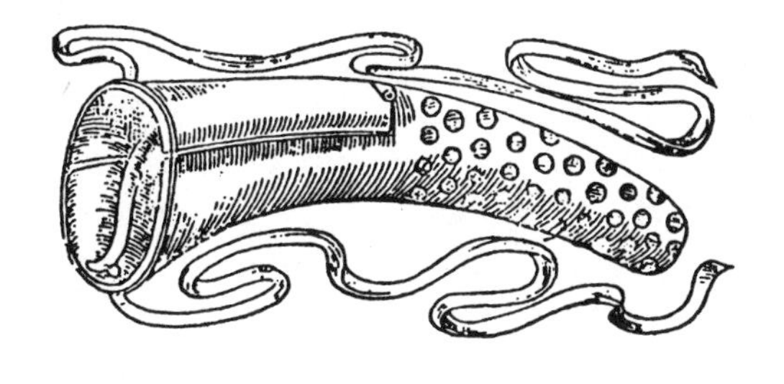
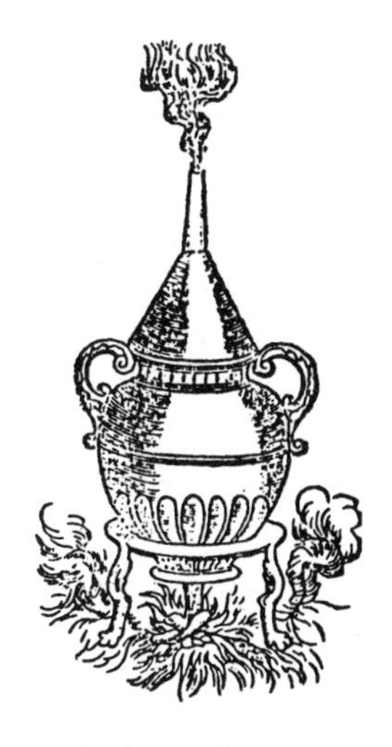

FIG. 9. Renaissance instruments for subfumigation. From Ambroise Paré, *L'opera ostetrico-ginecologica di Ambrogio Paré*, ed. Vittorio Pedore (Bologna: Cappelli, 1966), 166.

no such delicacy in 1889 when he described vulvular massage, including details of both internal and external manipulation with the fingers, in a work on electricity and massage.[9]

Although mechanisms of various kinds were available by the third quarter of the nineteenth century, not all advocates of physical therapies for hysteria endorsed them. George Massey, a well-known American physician who was actively involved in the development of electrotherapeutics, nonetheless considered "massage with the hand as the only efficient method" of treating hysterical women, "rejecting all machinery, muscle-beaters, etc., as either but poor substitutes for the hand of the *masseur* or as presenting an entirely different therapeutic measure."[10]

Silas Weir Mitchell, the rest-cure physician who has been identified as the antihero of Charlotte Perkins Gilman's *The Yellow Wallpaper*, was an advocate of massage; however, in 1877 he warned his fellow physicians that "the early use of massage is apt in some nervous women to cause increased nervousness and even loss of sleep," though "very soon the patient begins to find the massage soothing and to complain when it is omitted."[11] Mitchell may also have been the physician Thomas Low

Nichols referred to in his 1850 tract on the merits of the water cure for pregnant women:

> One man—if I do not too much insult humanity in giving him that appellation—residing in the vicinity of New York, has made these female diseases a specialty . . . The infamy of his bold quackeries and obscene manipulations would make the paper blush on which it was written. I have known of case after case which he has maltreated; and I know of no case in which, after a time, and when the peculiar excitement he induces has lost its effect, the patient has not sunk into a worse condition.[12]

Hydropathy and Hydrotherapy

Bathing of all kinds, but especially at spas or public bathing establishments, has been associated with sexuality in Western culture since antiquity.[13] Medicinal immersion in hot springs probably predates the fifth century B.C., and it was known in North America long before the arrival of Europeans. Native Americans are said to have discovered some of the hot springs and mineral springs on this continent by following the trails of animals that used them.[14] It was in Europe and Britain, and later in Europeanized America, that bathing spas acquired their reputation for luxury and dissipation. Gambling and beverages considerably stronger than mineral water were usually available at spas as alternatives to balneotherapy, or as entertainment for the companions of the afflicted.[15] Even the physicians were sometimes suspect: Francis Power Cobbe cast vague aspersions in 1881 on the morality of physicians who specialized in spa practice.[16] As late as the mid-twentieth century, Georges Simenon could plausibly suggest that gambling at spas counted as part of the therapy.[17] Iris Murdoch's novel *The Philosopher's Pupil* is set in the mythical bath town of Ennistone, which, according to the author, has a dark reputation for unmentionable vices.[18]

The Roman baths are reported to have been important venues for prostitution, a point to which an eighteenth-century German writer drew attention when he declared England's Bath and Tunbridge Wells the equals of the Caracalla in depravity.[19] Bath had by that time had a scandalous reputation for more than a hundred years. Despite (or perhaps because of) this infamy, British royalty gamely visited the place: Queen Anne in 1616 and Queen Catherine in 1663, the latter in search, significantly enough, of a cure for infertility.[20]

In Western Europe, long before the modern period, women went to mineral springs for such treatments as Catherine received at Bath.[21] Spas became fashionable even for the not very sick in Europe and Britain in the eighteenth century, and they reached fad proportions in the nineteenth. Tobias Smollett, who wrote an essay on the water cure in 1752, remarked that pumped water was good for "hysterical Disorders . . . Obstructions of the Menses, and all cases, where it is necessary to make a revulsion from the head, and to invite the juices downwards." He was an enthusiastic supporter of hydrotherapy in obstetrics as well, observing that "besides these uses of the Warm Bath, it is of great service in promoting delivery, by relaxing the part in those women who are turned of thirty before the first child; and in such as are naturally contracted in consequence of a rigid fibre, and robust constitution." He goes to commend a "Mr. Cleland, Surgeon" at Bath, who had proposed to the medical staff "a very ingenious apparatus he had contrived, for some complaints peculiar to the fair sex." Unfortunately, Smollett declines to describe this apparatus.[22]

The Austrian physician Vicenz Priessnitz is usually credited (or discredited) with making the water cure in the 1830s and 1840s what transcendental meditation was to the 1970s. The fashion for hydrotherapy in Europe, Britain, and the United States lasted more than half a century, probably because its pleasures, comforts, luxuries, and lack of medical discomfort so endeared it to patients and their companions.[23] At a time when about half of all surgical patients died either on the operating table or of complications afterward, physicians noted with interest (or on occasion indignation) that their clientele approached water cures with far less fear and repugnance than they did the measures of traditional "heroic medicine." Priessnitz seems to have been the first to systematically exploit the commercial advantages of this feature of hydrotherapy.

Even in Priessnitz's day there was an emphasis on women as patients. The Austrian technology, the first to be called "the douche," was simply cold water impelled by gravity, but both earlier and later methods used hot or warm pumped water. Priessnitz's cure, primitive as it was, was all the rage; his caseload grew from 45 in 1829 to 1,400 ten years later, with many patients coming from Britain and remote parts of Europe.[24] The famous Father Sebastien Kneipp, another European hydropath, set great store by the use of pumped water aimed at the pelvis as a treatment for female complaints.[25] In Europe the physicians themselves might operate the douche apparatus, but in the United States this was considered professionally dubious, and therapeutic assistants were usually employed. J. A. Irwin, for example, writing in 1892, had considerable faith in hydrotherapy, both as a therapeutic measure and as a prescription most patients were willing to take. Bathing in mineral waters, he said, had the advantage of "stimulating qualities of the gas and minerals, which are appreciated by the skin as a kind of textural unctuosity." He had reservations, however, about what he called "local irrigation" to relieve pelvic congestion in women, not because he thought it ineffective, but because he deemed it a threat to the decorum of the attending physician: patients stood in front of the doctor "receiving the column of water alternately, or as circumstances dictate, upon the spine and anterior surface of the body—a procedure somewhat startling to the Anglo-American sense of propriety, and scarcely in accord with our notions of professional dignity."[26]

R. J. Lane, who wrote about the English spa Malvern in 1851, quotes a male patient as saying that "the ladies are bolder-like with the wet sheets and Douches, and that, than the gentlemen." Malvern at this time used the Priessnitzian douche, a gravity-powered fall of water from a cistern eighteen feet overhead. Lane, evidently in awe of women's enthusiasm for the effects of hydrotherapy, mentions a lady who took the douche in the form of Niagara Falls, a sixty-foot fall at that point, and remarked, with some understatement, that "the Water Cure commends itself to the ladies." The douche, which he himself seems to have regarded with some trepidation, he reports as "so powerful a stimulant, that persons are frequently known, on coming out of the douche, to declare that they feel as much elation and buoyancy of spirits, as if they had been drinking champagne."[27] I shall have more to say about this elation later. Refinements were added as the century progressed. In 1867 the water cure at Matlock Bank in England had warm-water douche treatments for women plus electrotherapy and electric-bath installations. About 2,000 patients a year were treated there, of both sexes but with women predominating.

Another English spa of the second half of the nineteenth century provided horseback exercise, a traditional treatment for hysteria, to its women patients as an adjunct to hydrotherapy.[28] The companions and families of these patients often participated in the pleasures of the spa and its local service businesses.[29]

After therapeutic douches were installed at Bath in the 1880s, over 80,000 bathers converged on Britain's most famous spring to sample the latest hydriatic appliances.[30] Even the formerly disapproving traditional physicians were sometimes forced to give ground on the appeal of hydrotherapy to patients. W. B. Oliver, writing in the prestigious London medical journal *Lancet* in 1896, said of hydriatic massage that "the mechanical agency of percussion and vibration" of the water was modified by its temperature, so that when the jets of water strike the surface of the skin or "when it is applied in the form of a traveling douche accompanied by a vibratory form of massage, the vasomotor system is much more powerfully affected than by any form of still bathing."[31]

The douche was one of many therapies for hysteria in use at the Salpêtrière in the 1890s, when Freud was a visiting student there; Gilles de la Tourette reports that it was applied locally to the "hyperaesthetic" areas on the "front of the trunk."[32] Walter McClellan, who practiced hydrotherapy at Saratoga Springs in the early twentieth century, describes douche therapy as "a current of water directed against the surface or into a cavity of the body." He recommends supplies of both hot and cold water with a mixing valve, and a "hose or nozzle for projecting the stream of water onto the patient's skin," preferably one with enough pressure so that the water "may be projected from a distance of 10 to 15 feet."[33] Water at a lower pressure could be applied from the sides. Although McClellan's account is dated 1940, it is consistent with illustrations of the douche dating from the 1860s through the early twentieth century (see figs. 10, 11, and 12).[34]

Americans seized on the spa concept with their characteristic enthusiasm for marriages of health with luxury and good living. So convivial were nineteenth-century American spas that a good many of their visitors did not even pretend to an affliction.[35] Alexander MacKay wrote in the 1840s that "of the vast crowds who flock annually to Saratoga, but a small proportion are invalids."[36] Marietta Holley's 1887 *Samantha at Saratoga* does not even mention the baths, although perhaps Holley in-

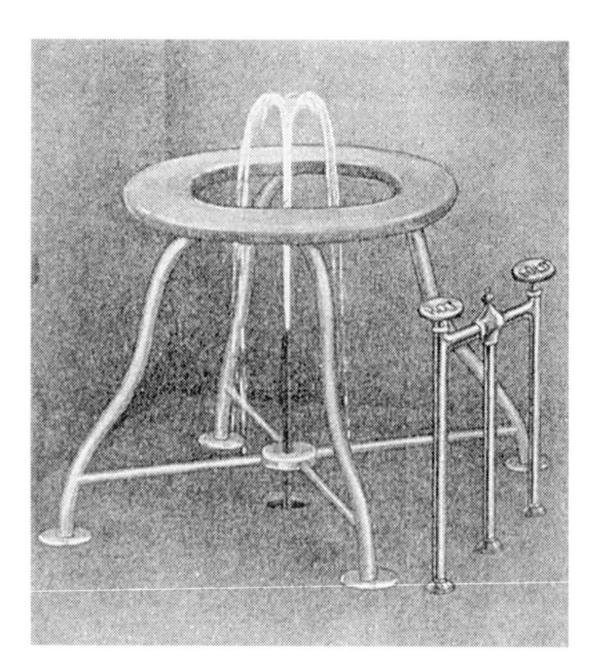

FIG. 10. The ascending douche at Saratoga, about 1900. From Guy Hinsdale, *Hydrotherapy* (Philadelphia: W. B. Saunders, 1910), 224.

tended to omit any reference to such questionable practices as douche therapy. Samantha and her companions primly drink water in the Pump Room, with all their fashionable clothes on, and admire their luxurious surroundings.[37]

Although Austria claims credit for commercializing hydrotherapy in the nineteenth century, there is considerable evidence that American spas were thriving even before Priessnitz initiated his famous medical entrepreneurship. The travel author James Stuart said that "fifteen hundred people have been known to arrive in a week" at the spas at Saratoga and Ballston Springs, New York.[38] Hot mineral springs, however odoriferous, were the most popular, but even cold-water springs repaid hydropathic entrepreneurship.[39] New York State was a leader in the nineteenth-century spa industry, with a reported one-third of all United States water cures in 1847.[40] Saratoga remained New York's most fashionable water cure until the early years of the twentieth century, with its added attractions of a nationally famous racetrack and casino. The town also had, by the 1860s, a remarkably dense population of physicians, some of whom, like J. A. Irwin, made international reputations for themselves in hydrotherapy.[41]

Women were the most visible, and probably the most profitable, patients at these establishments.[42] At Round Hill Water-Cure Retreat, for example, Halsted used Taylor mechanisms in treating chronic diseases of women to produce "statuminating vitalizing motion." The New Hygienic Institute in New York City advertised in 1858 "the Swedish Movement Cure, Turkish baths, electric baths, vapor baths, water-cure, machine vibrations, lifting cure, magnetism and healthful food." At some spas the patient's circulation was stimulated by flogging with wet towels or sheets.[43] Writing of these establishments in 1984, historian Kathryn

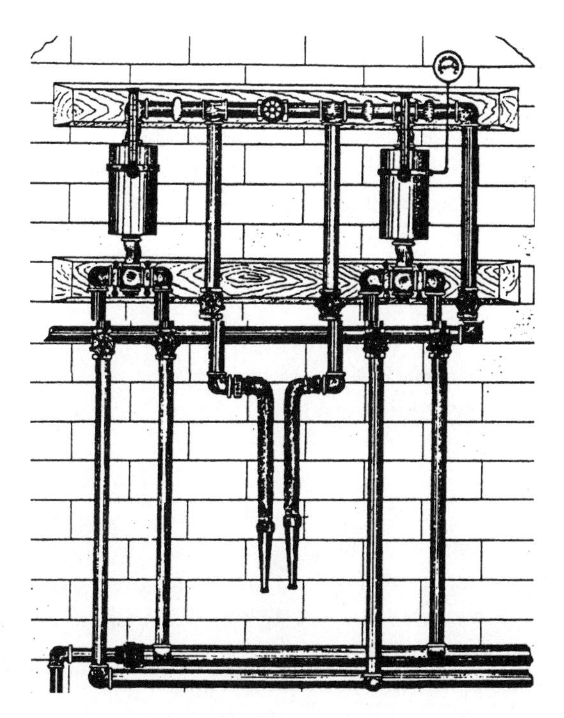

FIG. 11. Pope model of douche equipment, about 1900. From Curran Pope, *Practical Hydrotherapy: A Manual for Students and Practitioners* (Cincinnati: Lancet-Clinic, 1909).

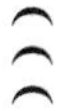

Sklar asserted that "sexual release through genital stimulation was a rudimentary water cure experience for women."[44]

From Ballston Springs (now Ballston Spa), New York, near the famous springs at Saratoga, we have the journal of a young woman, Abigail May, who eventually died of the disease (probably cancer) for which she had gone to the spa. The water cure seems to have brightened her last illness, however, despite the constant pain she suffered, although it had no curative effect. She says of her first encounter with the douche that it was difficult to summon the courage, but that "taking care to have laudanum handy" she took the plunge. After the initial shock, "I scream'd merrily—so says Mama—for my own part I do not remember much about it—I felt finely for two hours after bathing."[45] She went to the baths again on a Sunday with a friend, an experience of which she says that "I was so much pleased with the Bath that probably I staid in too long—for immediately on returning to the house I was sensible of feeling extremely weak and languid."[46]

Elation followed by drowsiness were frequently observed in douche and massage patients. Simon Baruch wrote in 1897 that the douche was "the most stimulating of all hydriatic applications" and went to say that "it is not necessary to dwell upon the fact that every physiological indication is fulfilled by the douche. The nerve centers are aroused, the respiration is deepened, the circulation is invigorated, the secretions are increased." He was especially enthusiastic about the results of "douches upon the loins" in cases of hysteria and neurasthenia.[47] Edward Johnson, who thought that hysterics should have douche treatment every day for a month, remarked that even this intensive treatment regimen did not satisfy all of his patients, and that he experienced "difficulty . . . in keeping them within rational limits. As soon as they become sensible of decided improvement, they become enthusiastic—they think they can never have enough—that the more they get, the faster they will get well." He describes his patients' enthusiasm for the douche, "generally looked upon as the 'lion' of every hydropathic establishment," and remarks that this type of treatment is the one most often recommended to friends: "so many pleasant marvels to recount at home, and to excite the wondering curiosity of friends and relations."[48] Johnson seems here to attribute the exciting effects of the douche to a kind of hydriatic equivalent of a roller-coaster ride. Mary Louise Shew, who warned or perhaps promised women that hydrotherapeutic methods would produce new and unexpected sensations, quoted Johnson's description of douche patients in 1844, where he reports "the most intense impression which can be made by the application of cold water." Women are advised that "it sometimes produces the most extraordinary effects, as weeping, laughing, trembling, &tc."[49]

Mary Gove Nichols wrote that the douche "is a very exciting application, acting powerfully upon the whole system," recommended as a way of reducing congestion caused by "excessive indulgence of amativeness," in the form of either intercourse or masturbation.[50] According to Nichols, the hydriatic douche restored tone and vigor to the female reproductive system. Her husband, Thomas Low Nichols, after discussing the many virtues of hydrotherapy as a general treatment, asserts that "there is one class of diseases to which the adaptation of the Water-Cure ought every where to be known, and no false delicacy will atone to my conscience for not giving them the prominence they deserve. I allude to the diseases of women." He discusses the relative merits of inpatient and outpatient therapy, mentioning that his establishment serves women who come in only for "[wet-sheet] packs and douches" and notes that "coming from the douche, a patient feels like jumping over fences."[51] James Manby Gully, a contemporary of the Nicholses, recommended the douche for "nervous headache" in women, which he considered one of the hysteroneurasthenic disorders. Gully liked to stimulate the spine with the jet of water first, then zero in on locations like "the loins."[52]

William H. Dieffenbach, an early twentieth-century advocate of hydriatic methods, endorsed a combination of hydrotherapy with manual massage and vibratory treatment, especially for hysteria and neurasthenia, which like his predecessors he considered related disorders. He thought that "conjugal incompatibility, sexual excess, masturbation, sexual continence, habits of over-indulgence in coffee, tea, tobacco, drugs and alcoholic beverages" contributed to neurasthenia and hysteria.[53] Apparently the etiological paradigm could accommodate either too much sex or too little, a theory quite appropriate to a treatment that produced orgasms perhaps not regularly achieved in conjugal expressions of "amativeness." His contemporary Curran Pope also thought that applying the douche to the "inner surface of the thighs" was an effective treatment of the sequelae of "imperfect or unsatisfactory intercourse."[54] Pope waxed even more poetic than his colleagues on the merits of the douche in achieving patients' compliance with therapy: "Douches are, as a rule, more agreeable to the majority of individuals than the other forms of hydriatic procedure . . . It sets the tissues in a vibration impossible to describe; experienced, it is never forgotten." As far as Pope was concerned, the douche was unparalleled as a tonic. "Administered at high or low temperatures, under a strong pressure, it is capable of arousing the most sluggish and intolerant function of the body." In melancholia, neurasthenia, hysteria, and "other nervous affections, there is no weapon equal to the douche in restorative power."[55] Guy Hinsdale at the same period thought that menopausal women were especially good candidates for hydriatic treatment. "The asthenic physical condition," he wrote, "the mental depression, the irritability, the nervousness, and especially the sleeplessness, are certainly relieved to a great extent by a judicious use of these carbonated saline baths."[56]

The reported enthusiasm of women for the douche is not surprising. A jet of pumped water aimed at the male genitalia is more likely to produce pain than pleasure, but the use of water as a female masturbatory method is well documented, although in this century it is apparently employed only by a minority. Shere Hite reported in 1976 that about 2 percent of her respondents masturbated with water, using either the direct force of the water from the tap or hand-held shower hoses.[57] Linda Wolfe's *Cosmo Report* of 1981 also mentioned this technique.[58] This method of masturbation raises questions about the early popularity of such hoses at the beginning of this century, when bathtubs first became common in urban households.[59] Donald Greydanus, who cites W. R. Miller and H. I. Lief's estimates that masturbation is practiced by 97 percent of males and 78 percent of females, mentions "tap water masturbation" but provides no further data on its incidence.[60] In a popular anthology of women's fantasies published in 1975, the speed and efficacy with which a jet of pumped water produces orgasm in women is noted in a chapter called "Playtime in the Pool."[61] Inspired by a mention of masturbation with water in the first edition of *Our Bodies, Our Selves* in 1970, Eugene Halpert reported on this practice to the American Psychoanalytic Association in 1973, using three case studies of his own female patients. A staunch Freudian, Halpert makes it clear from the beginning that he considers this behavior aberrant: in each of the three cases, he

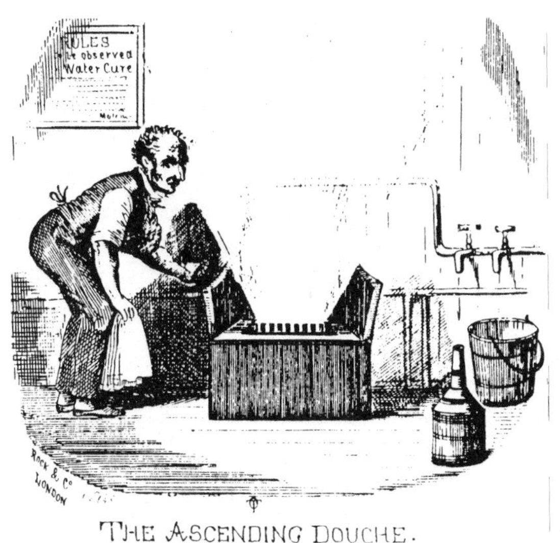
RULES
to be observed
Water Cure
Rock & Co
London
THE ASCENDING DOUCHE.
"Now Sir, please to take a seat here."

FIG. 12. British male reaction to the ascending douche, from Joseph Buckley, *Recollections of the Late John Smedley and the Water Cure* (1888; Matlock, England: Arkwright Society, 1973).

asserts that the patient "was frigid" in the context of intercourse. After the obligatory review of the literature and a brief discussion of male masturbation with water, he describes the phenomenon reported by his three patients: "They all used the identical method, lying on their backs in the tub and positioning themselves so that the water from the faucet could be run on their genitals." Adjustments in the temperature and flow of water onto the clitoris were usually necessary, after which orgasm reliably occurred in short order. Halpert, after dutifully describing what he takes to be relevant dreams, fantasies, and childhood experiences of the three women, concludes that these women are fulfilling fantasies to the effect that "I have my father's penis and can urinate/ejaculate like a man, and I am able to urinate and destroy/castrate with my powerful stream in revenge for castration."[62] Apparently, to a Freudian the production of orgasm in this manner required an elaborate explanation beyond the straightforward desire for pleasure and sexual release.[63]

Electrotherapeutic devices were an invention of the eighteenth century, beginning with electrostatic generators that transferred static electricity to the hands and progressing, in the nineteenth century, to various kinds of direct-current devices and electrets.[64] The latter, such as "electric" hairbrushes and corsets, lacked any power source; their presumed efficacy consisted in the electrical charging of the materials during their manufacture.[65] In the mid-nineteenth century, electric current from batteries, including so-called "vibrators" (actually inductive devices that rhythmically interrupted the current), were used to control dental pain.[66] Audrey Davis says that subsequent developments included "a spectacular range of devices . . . for applying heat, electricity, water, x-rays, and various motions and vibrations to the body in the period beginning at the end of the nineteenth century."[67]

In the second half of the nineteenth century and the early part of the twentieth, there was considerable medical and scientific interest in electrolytes, human skin conductivity, and the effects of electrical stimulation on the health of plants and animals.[68] Some doctors thought that electrical contraction of muscles could be useful as a substitute for exercise.[69] Of particular interest to physicians was the perceived potential of electrotherapeutic treatment of impotence and "sexual debility" in men, both thought to be caused at least in part by masturbation.[70] Popular medical literature and advertising encouraged men's anxiety about losing virility to the solitary vice, and thousands of electrical devices were sold directly to consumers on the strength of their alleged ability to restore masculine powers; some physicians specialized in providing electrotherapeutic services.[71] Richard von Krafft-Ebing mentions these devices briefly, citing a case of a young man who masturbated with a battery. Arousal to orgasm in this fashion would certainly have convinced purchasers that their male powers were in a healthy condition.[72] Historian of medicine David Reynolds remarks on the phenomenon:

> It was perhaps inevitable that finally, at about the time of Freud's initial papers on the sexual bases of neurosis, Rousell should report "It is especially in the genital organs that electricity is truly marvelous. Impotence disappears, strength and desire of youth return, and the man, old before his time,

> whether by excesses or privations, with the aid of electric fustigation, can become fifteen years younger." Electrotherapeutic currents were also recommended for nymphomania. Presumably the treatment for nymphomania differed from that for impotency—perhaps a reversal of polarity. The responsibility of the nineteenth century physician in treating impotency and nymphomania with electricity was awesome. A mix-up in the leads could result in personal tragedy in one patient—a social menace in another.[73]

William Snowdon Hedley wrote in 1892 about a set of therapeutic procedures known as "hydro-electrization," which included an "electric douche" applied with saline "water electrodes." The method was recommended as a stimulant for "heightening cutaneous sensibility and quickening motor excitability."[74] In 1903 the International Correspondence Schools' *System of Electrotherapeutics* recommended an electric douche regimen that combined electrical currents with hydrotherapeutic and sometimes vibratory or manual massage.[75] By 1918 manufacturers of physical therapy equipment, like Kellogg in Battle Creek, Michigan, were producing apparatus that would provide alternating current through a hydroelectric bath, utilizing a "motor-operated magneto."[76]

As Reynolds indicates, electrotherapeutic methods were used in women's disorders as well as men's, including not only the nymphomania he mentions but also dysmenorrhea, infertility, "frigidity," and that turn-of-the-century bane of the educated classes, neurasthenia.[77] Richard Cowen wrote in 1900 that electricity worked well in dysmenorrhea when combined with local massage to "stimulate the circulation in the pelvic organs, to get rid of the congestion and the hyperaemia."[78] Herman Hoyd endorsed battery application of "faradic current" by the patient herself to improve uterine and vaginal muscle tone.[79] A. Lapthorn Smith, writing in Horatio Bigelow's 1894 textbook of electrotherapeutics, advocated the use of battery faradization in amenorrhea and female infertility, despite the technical difficulties of keeping the batteries filled, charged, and ready for use. Bigelow had "always been reluctant to apply local treatment to unmarried women" but considered it appropriate for wives. He could, he said, "testify positively" to visible results in amenorrhea and infertility, "but with regard to the development of any passion I cannot speak very decidedly, as it is difficult to induce women to speak much about it," although in a few cases he felt he had "reason to believe that

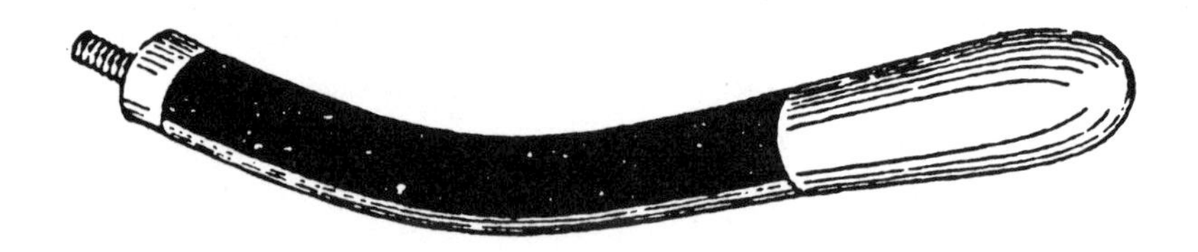

FIG. 13. Vaginal electrode, from Franklin Benjamin Gottschalk, *Practical Electro-therapeutics, with a Special Section on Vibratory Stimulation* (Hammond, Ind.: F. S. Betz, 1903).

sexual feeling actually was experienced after many years of married life without it."[80]

Franklin H. Martin wrote in 1892 about electrical treatment of "nervous inefficiency" in women, brought on by childbearing, "excessive cohabitation, or undue treatment of a local variety." In his view the "nervous perversion" he saw in his patients was more often due to "too much studying" and "the worries of motherhood" than to the masturbation his colleagues suspected as the etiology.[81] Martin described his procedure as "a process of kneading or petrisage . . . performed over the surface of the body, dwelling particularly on the motor points of the muscles, in which the current is simply strong enough to produce an agreeable prickling sensation."[82]

Havelock Ellis, writing between 1897 and 1910 on "auto-erotism," seems convinced that mild electric shocks produce sexual arousal in women. In his discussion of what he calls *rin-no-tama,* what we would now call ben-wa balls for vaginal insertion, he says that the movement of such devices "and the resulting vibration produces a prolonged voluptuous titillation, a gentle shock as from a weak electric inductive apparatus,"[83] throwing possible light on the use of electricity to awaken or reawaken desire.

John Harvey Kellogg, who was a great believer in the benefits of pelvic muscle contractions for treating neurasthenic women, told attendees of the International Electrical Congress in 1904 that galvanic electrical methods achieved spectacular results when applied to the genital area:

> The contraction is spasmodic rather than tetanic in character, as when the faradic current is employed. By proper adjustment of the current, strong muscular contractions may be induced without producing the slightest sensation on the skin, and without any pain sensation whatever. With one electrode placed in the rectum or the vagina, and the other upon the abdomen, strong contractions of the abdominal muscles may be produced, and even of the muscles of the upper thigh, without any sensation other than that of motion. I have frequently seen patients, while receiving the current in this manner, shaking so vigorously under its influence that the office table was made to tremble quite violently with the movement.[84]

Electrotherapeutic devices sold to consumers for self-treatment seem to have enjoyed significant popularity between about 1880 and the late 1910s (figs. 13 and 14). One of these was the Butler Electro-massage Machine of 1888, pictured in figure 2 (chapter 1), which combined roller massage with a mild electrical shock. For uterine diseases, the roller was to be used "over lower abdomen, from 10 to 15 minutes. Change the treatment every other day, using the vaginal sponge-electrode, and applying roller over lower abdomen ten minutes, and lower spine five minutes." Butler expressed his conviction that three-quarters of the female population suffered from conditions for which his massage device was indicated. Among the many testimonials that appear in his advertising is one from a grateful husband, who reports that his wife treated herself for "female weakness, and general debility of the system, with the most gratifying results."[85]

Eight years earlier, Butler had been marketing his device primarily to professionals, recommending it for "nervous exhaustion," for which massage upward from the feet, first gently and then kneading until "the skin [is] made thoroughly red." He describes patient responses not unlike those reported for hydrotherapy: "The immediate effect of the treatment on these nervous patients, is that of a calmative; they seem infinitely relieved of something; what—they seem unable to describe. They often want to sleep."[86] This device, Butler asserted, could be used by the patient herself "after a lesson or two"; by 1888 he seemed to perceive no need for professional intervention at any point.[87] Another home device manufactured by a New York City firm about 1900 was recommended to purchasers interested in "developing and hardening the bust"[88] (fig. 15).

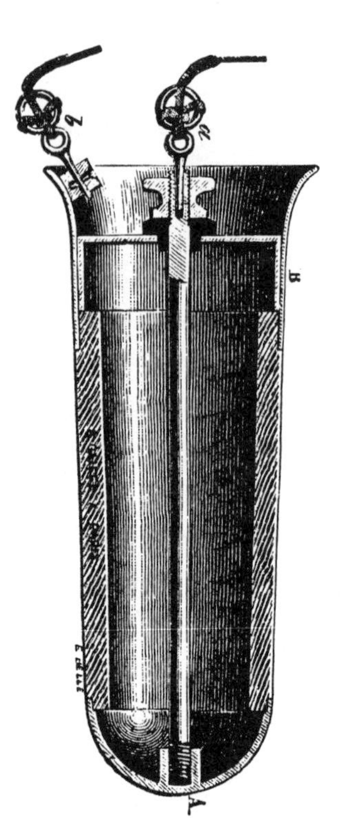

FIG. 14. "Excitateur vulvo-uterin" electrode, a faradization electrode illustrated in Auguste Élisabeth Philogène Tripier, *Leçons cliniques sur les maladies de femmes: Thérapeutique générale et applications de l'électricité à ces maladies* (Paris: Octave Doin, 1883).

The Electrical Building at the Columbian Exposition in Chicago in 1893 had an exhibition of electromedical devices, "Group 135" of the many new applications of electric power.[89]

Physicians had mixed feelings about electromedical apparatus; John Girdner in *Munsey's* of April 1903 quotes "a distinguished specialist" as saying that "at present medical electricity occupies a humbler position in applied therapeutics than it deserves" and goes on to say that "there are so many quacks and charlatans who deceive and rob the public by promises to cure disease with one electrical device or another that the medical profession is disposed to look askance at all such claims."[90] John

Shoemaker, writing in 1907, seems to have had similarly grave reservations about electrotherapeutic devices in the hands of the unscrupulous. He says that electricity combined with massage, exercise, and good diet can be a useful regimen in some maladies, but that "without such therapeutic accessories, electricity, like massage, is very restricted in its usefulness and tends toward charlatanism."[91]

Electrical massage machinery was available to physicians from reputable suppliers like William H. Armstrong and Company of Indianapolis, which in 1901 manufactured both electrical rollers and a "portable combination massage instrument" called an "electro-spatteur" with a "vibrating fork" between the massage rollers.[92] Electrotherapeutic suppliers who sold equipment primarily to physicians were much less flamboyant in their advertising claims than consumer companies, and perhaps for this reason they retained their respectable medical reputation into the twentieth century.[93]

Despite the odor of quackery that had begun to cling to electrotherapeutic devices for self-treatment by the late 1880s, they continued to be widely advertised and sold. The *Census of Manufactures* for 1905 noted that electrotherapeutic apparatus worth more than a million dollars was manufactured "in no fewer than 66 establishments, chiefly in Illinois and New York," at a time when the total value of electrical household goods produced was about a fifth of this figure.[94] By 1914 the United States production of electrotherapeutic equipment was valued at more than $2.6 million.[95] As late as 1947, after X-ray equipment had been reclassified out of the category, "electro-therapeutic apparatus" was valued in the *Census* at $7.6 million.[96] These statistics were not, however, disaggregated by sales to consumers versus those to physicians, and figures were not provided on the number of units represented by the total values of manufactured goods. Clearly, the questionable character of these devices did not interfere significantly with sales.

The United States Battery Agency, for example, advertised in 1889 in *Dorcas Magazine*, to an almost exclusively female readership of embroiderers and other needle artisans, "All Physicians Agree that every family should have an Electric Battery in their house." In the illustration, electrodes for every conceivable bodily orifice are depicted as accessories to the device.[97] Less ambitious was the Oxydonor of 1902, a "hydro-electrization" device for the home that had the additional adver-

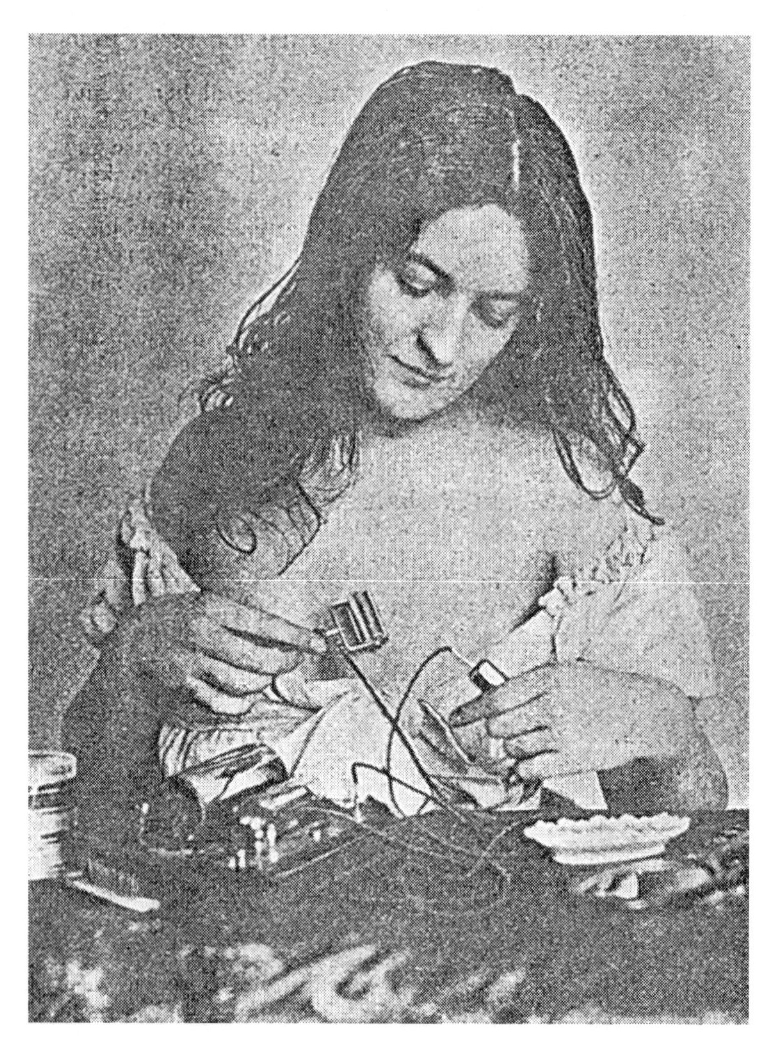

Fig. 15. "Developing and hardening the bust" with electricity, about 1900.

tised feature of adding healthful qualities to the air by producing ozone.[98] Instant beauty for women and restoration of head hair to men were among the miracles attributed to home electromedical devices by their advertisements.[99] Violet ray devices, which used electricity merely to generate light and heat in their brilliant purple electrodes, were report-

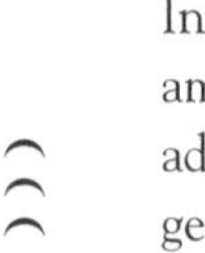

edly less startling than "faradization" in their effects on the patient. The advertising stated that "a huge voltage of electricity is obtained and applied to the body or hair but without any shock whatever, and the only sensation being a pleasant warmth."[100] Like the electric battery described in *Dorcas*, the violet ray came with a formidable set of attachments appropriate to the various orifices, and some of them combined vibratory capabilities and ozone generation with the allegedly therapeutic effects of violet light. One of these was made by Lindstrom, a vibrator manufacturer, and marketed in *Popular Mechanics* as an analgesic device, presumably to a mostly male readership.[101]

Mechanical Massagers and Vibrators

Soon after train travel became a standard feature of industrialized life in the nineteenth century, it became the focus of an iatromachy over whether it was good or bad for women, primarily because it subjected them to vibration.[102] As we have seen, many physicians of earlier centuries thought the vibration of horseback riding and carriages benefited hysterics: Soranus, Paré, Sydenham, and others prescribed rocking, riding, and even dancing in addition to massage or marriage.[103] Charles Meigs in 1854 recommended that women enhance their "pelvic determination" of blood by "galloping on horseback, which powerfully develops it."[104] Krafft-Ebing and George Beard both reported that some of their male patients were aroused to orgasm by equitation, and historians John Haller and Robin Haller report that horseback riding was one of the nineteenth-century treatments for impotence.[105] The movement of a railroad car clearly provided a similar but perhaps more intense experience of the same kind.[106] Predictably, this enhanced intensity was applauded by some physicians and deplored by others as a kind of overdose of physical therapy, which was thought to produce arousal or orgasm in women travelers. Charles Malchow thoughtfully provided directions on the posture most conducive to achieving this effect in a work that by 1923 had gone through six editions and twenty-seven printings. After noting that riding in vibrating vehicles such as railway carriages "sometimes occasions excitement, especially when sitting so as to be leaning forward" and could produce sexual arousal in women, he warns that "riding a bicycle or run-

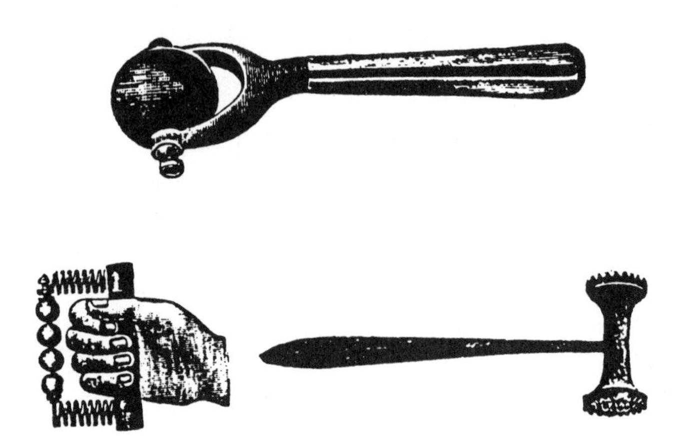

Fig. 16. Nineteenth-century muscle beaters.

ning a sewing machine tends, by the movements of the lower limbs and the friction occasioned, to sometimes produce such a condition of the genital organs as to lead to excitement and even orgasm."[107]

He was not alone in expressing concern about the vibration and thigh rubbing associated with the use of pedal-operated sewing machines.[108] Later in the century, some physicians suspected that bicycles overstimulated women in the same way.[109] Haller and Haller tell us that "a physician from Tennessee reported that one of his patients took up the bicycle for the purpose of masturbation and admitted to him that 'it was no uncommon thing . . . to experience a sexual orgasm three or four times on a ride of one hour.'"[110] Robert William Taylor, who wrote *A Practical Treatise on Sexual Disorders of the Male and Female* at the turn of the century, was convinced that horseback riding, sewing machines, and bicycles all encouraged masturbation in women.[111] We know little about how and how often nineteenth-century women masturbated, but there is more than ample documentary evidence that their male physicians expended considerable mental energy on the subject.

Russell Thacher Trall, a hydropathic physician and a colleague of John Harvey Kellogg, wrote in 1863 of the importance of physical therapies in diseases of women, which he said were otherwise very difficult to treat: "They are confessedly the *opprobrium medicorum* of the Profession, although not less than three-quarters of the business of modern physicians is in prescribing for them." For these ailments, Trall recommends "walking, dancing, jumping the rope, horseback riding &c" as active exercises, with "carriage-riding, rubbing and kneading the abdominal muscles" as "examples of appropriate passive exercise."[112]

Jean-Martin Charcot at the Salpêtrière, in the latter half of the nineteenth century, was one of the endorsers of rail travel for hysteroneurasthenic disorders and is said to have sent some of his patients on long trips over rough trackbeds for their health. He and his colleagues, however, eventually hit on the idea of shaking their patients in place, with various devices ranging from vibrating helmets to jolting chairs.[113] A number of variations on this theme were eventually devised, including chairs on springs that the patient operated by pulling two side levers (see fig. 17) and an electrical attachment for a rocking chair patented by Charles E. Hartelius in 1893, in which the rocking motion sent an electrical current through the patient.[114] John Harvey Kellogg's Good Health catalog of therapeutic appliances in 1909 offered physicians a vibratory chair, a vibrating bar, a trunk-shaking apparatus (like those used today in weight-loss studios), apparatus for percussion and mechanical kneading, and a very impressive electromechanical "centrifugal vibrator."[115]

Chairs and trunk shakers, however, were of little value when local treatment was indicated. Joseph Mortimer Granville, father of the modern electromechanical vibrator, briefly summarizes the history of his invention and includes an illustration of a spring-driven wind-up "percuteur" (fig. 18).[116] A device called the "concussor," available by 1898, was operated by foot power. Friedrich Bilz describes a device with a flywheel on a vertical stand, set in motion by a foot pedal (fig. 19). The business end is attached to "a so-called flexible axle (spiral spring) which can be easily twined in all directions." The vibratode "can easily be taken off and replaced by one of a different shape; it is provided with a ball joint just beyond the excentric [*sic*] bend, on which variously shaped end pieces or instruments made of guttapercha or ebony are fitted." Bilz notes with approval that "up to 3000 vibrations in a minute can be produced by rapid movement of the treadle by means of this machine, but an expert masseur cannot exceed 350 in the same length of time."[117] The foot-pedal device he describes was clearly the low-budget model; Bilz's own clinic had an electrically powered concussor. Mary Lydia H. A. Snow illustrates a different model of foot-powered vibrator, the "Victor,"

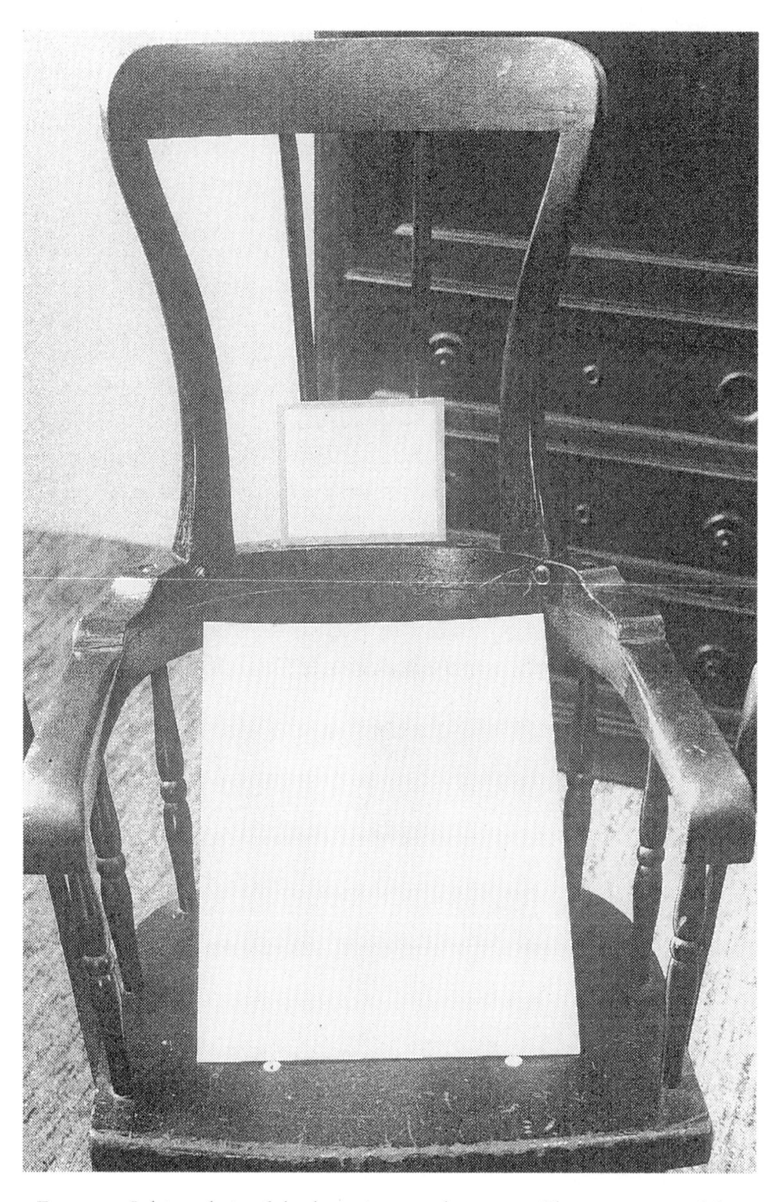

Fig. 17. Jolting chair of the late nineteenth century. Photo courtesy of the Potsdam Public Museum.

in her 1904 book on vibratory treatment. Vibrators operated only with human energy proved fairly persistent in the market. Versions of them were sold to consumers in the United States after 1900, and Schall and Son, medical instrument makers of London and Glasgow, were still offering human-powered vibrators to physicians in 1925.[118] Snow also discusses and depicts water-powered and pneumatic vibrators, both of which were later to become consumer products.

The latter half of the nineteenth century was also, as we observed in chapter 1, the era of the steam-powered vibrator. The Swedish physical therapist Gustaf Zander's European equipment for therapeutic exercise was the model for most spa machinery between 1860 and 1890; George Taylor improved on Zander's ideas as well as those of other physical therapy equipment inventors by attaching his "Medical Rubbing Apparatus" to a stationary steam engine.[119] Taylor received patents in 1869, 1872, 1876, and 1882 for various kinds of massage machinery.[120] He especially recommended his devices for "pelvic hyperaemia" in women, noting that its "vibration may be compared to the blows of an infinitesimal hammer, under continuous and very rapid action."[121] Of the hyperemia, he observed in his 1883 *Health for Women* that "rapid vibratory motion applied to the affected part and to the surrounding region, produces absorption and the reduction of enlargement in a remarkable and . . . satisfactory degree."[122]

Instrumental Prestige in the Vibratory Operating Room

Alphonso Rockwell reports that electromechanical vibrators were first used in medicine in 1878, at that nineteenth-century Mecca of physical therapies, the Salpêtrière in Paris. Significantly, their first use was on hysterical women.[123] Some controversy must have been associated with this practice, since the English physician and inventor Joseph Mortimer Granville, in his 1883 book on vibratory therapy, seems somewhat defensive about the issue:

> I should here explain that, with a view to eliminate possible sources of error in the study of these phenomena, I have never yet percussed a female

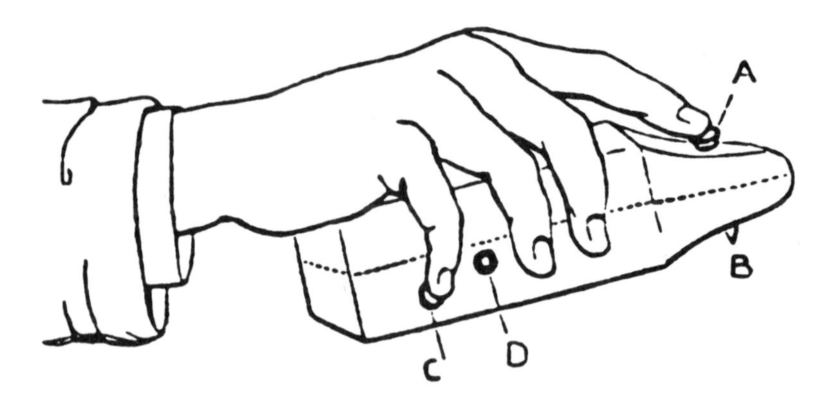

FIG. 18. Clockwork "percuteur," from Joseph Mortimer Granville, *Nerve-Vibration and Excitation as Agents in the Treatment of Functional Disorders and Organic Disease* (London: J. and A. Churchill, 1883).

> patient [with a vibrator], and have not founded any of my conclusions on the treatment of hysterical males. This is a matter of much moment in my judgment, and I am, therefore, careful to place the fact on record. I have avoided, and shall continue to avoid, the treatment of women by percussion, simply because I do not want to be hoodwinked, and help to mislead others, by the vagaries of the hysterical state or the characteristic phenomena of mimetic disease.[124]

Mortimer Granville's vibrator was powered by a large and heavy but allegedly portable battery and was equipped with a suitable array of vibratodes (fig. 20). It was manufactured to the physician's specifications by Weiss, a reputable British maker of medical instruments.[125] Mortimer Granville asserts his priority in the invention, although Felix Henri Boudet claimed this honor for Vigouroux of the Salpêtrière.

As I described in chapter 1, dozens of models of vibrators were available by 1900, using a variety of power sources, many with impressive sets of attachments.[126] There was a brief rash of publications on the subject, advocating the use of "vibrotherapy" for a variety of ailments in women and men, including arthritis, constipation, amenorrhea, inflammations, and tumors.[127] At English and French hospitals in Serbia, some wounded World War I soldiers received vibrotherapy.[128]

Physicians were advised to purchase professional-looking equipment, which could not be confused with consumer models. As Wallian observed in 1906 of the large number of vibrators available to physicians and the public: "The idea has been so vulgarized that the department stores and sporting goods houses are advertising 'Health' vibrators for home use." Wallian has nothing but scorn for these devices; professional machines with sophisticated vibratodes such as the fluid cushion applicators of the "Physician's Vibragenitant" were recommended (fig. 21).[129] Alfred Covey, author of *Profitable Office Specialities*, advised doctors in 1912 to invest in a good vibrator; prices ranged from $15 to $75.[130] In 1914 Wappler Electric offered an office model for $95 and a portable vibrator for $45; Manhattan Electrical Supply had a less costly line ranging from $25 to $40 at about the same time.[131] The elegant 125-pound Chattanooga Vibrator illustrated in figure 4 (chapter 1) sold for $200 in 1904 and was positioned, in modern marketing parlance, as a professional medical instrument, not a "massage machine." The company was careful to reassure prospective customers that "it is sold only to Physicians, and constructed for the express purpose of exciting the various organs of the body into activity through their central nerve supply."[132] Catalog illustrations show treatment of both sexes, including treatment of males through the rectum (fig. 22). The company assured prospective purchasers that "this instrument will be found to be an invaluable aid to the physician in the treatment of all nervous diseases and female troubles," later adding that "in cases where the patient is a woman and the nervousness is caused by either the ovaries or uterus, particular attention should be given to the lower part of the spine and also to the affected organs themselves."[133]

Franklin Gottschalk advised his fellow physicians in 1903 that the equipment should be carefully selected and maintained. He recommended that doctors acquire "at least two adjustable vibrators," one for slow massages of "fifty to one hundred fifty periods per minute, giving muscles time to rest between each alternate contraction," and another "for sedation, with a rapid vibration, adjustable for seven to nine thousand periods per minute." Gottschalk thought his techniques especially useful in menopause.[134]

In 1917 Anthony Matijaca commended vibrators to the readers of his *Principles of Electro-medicine, Electro-surgery and Radiology* as the

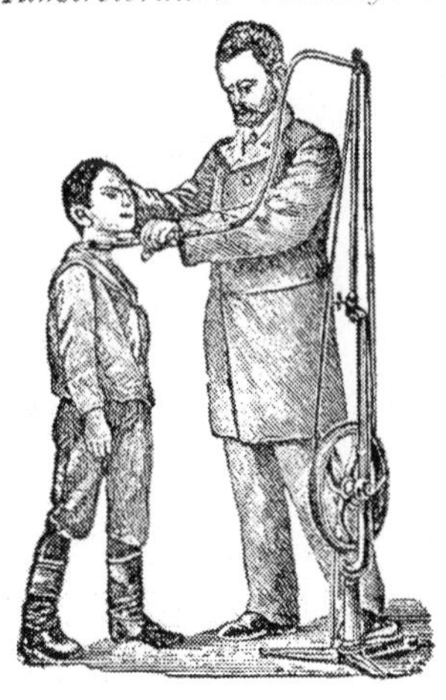

Massage apparatus
concussor.
Illust. vibration of the larynx.

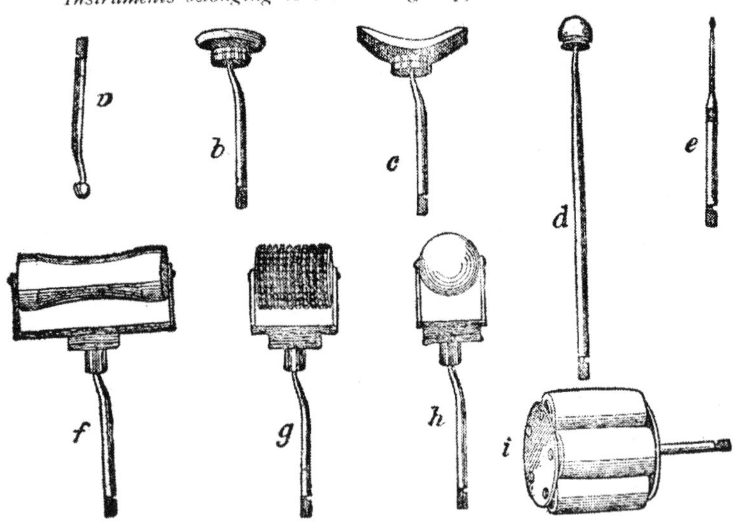

Fig. 19. Foot-powered vibrator with attachments, 1898.

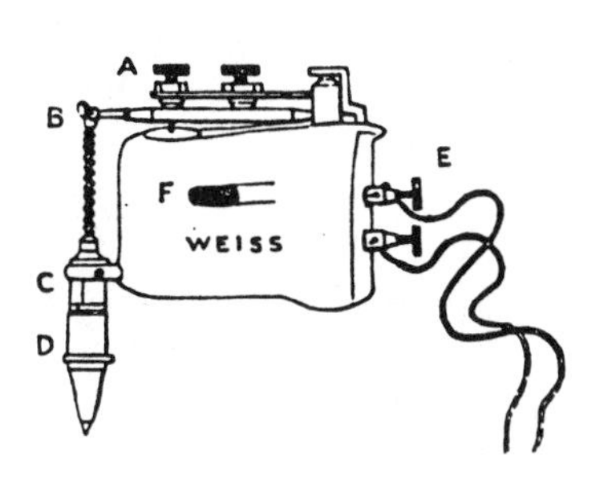

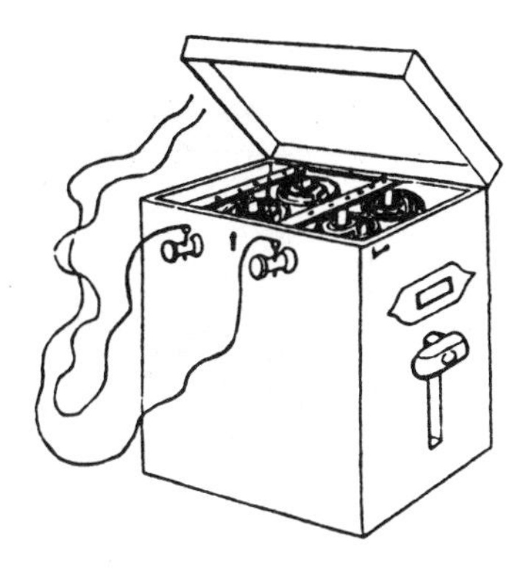

FIG. 20. Mortimer Granville's battery-powered vibrator, manufactured by Weiss, 1883.

only instrument of "mechano-therapy . . . which accomplishes something which cannot be accomplished by any other means." Apparently losing control of his spelling as he warmed to his subject, he enthused, "No human hand is capable of cummunicating [*sic*] to the tissues such rapid, steady and prolonged vibrations, and certain kneading and percussion movements, as the vibrator."[135]

The vibrator did not lack for theoreticians at the turn of the century. The most eloquent was Samuel Spencer Wallian, who wrote a series of articles for the *Medical Brief* in 1905, titled "The Undulatory Theory in Therapeutics." In the first paper he informs readers that all life is based on vibration, a principle that was to be echoed in popular advertising for home vibrators. The "variation in vibratory velocity," as he expressed it, produced various results in the great scheme of things: "A certain rate begets a *vermis*, another and higher rate produces a *viper*, a vertebrate, a *vestryman*" (emphasis in the original).[136]

His second paper concentrates on more practical issues, particularly the usefulness of vibrators in increasing the blood supply of the areas they were applied to. He argues that manual massage will do the same but "requires the expenditure of much time and strength on the part of the operator, and has practically no influence over deep-seated nerve or trophic centers."[137] Some of the more metaphysical components of Wallian's comments apparently resonated (as it were) with other philosoph-

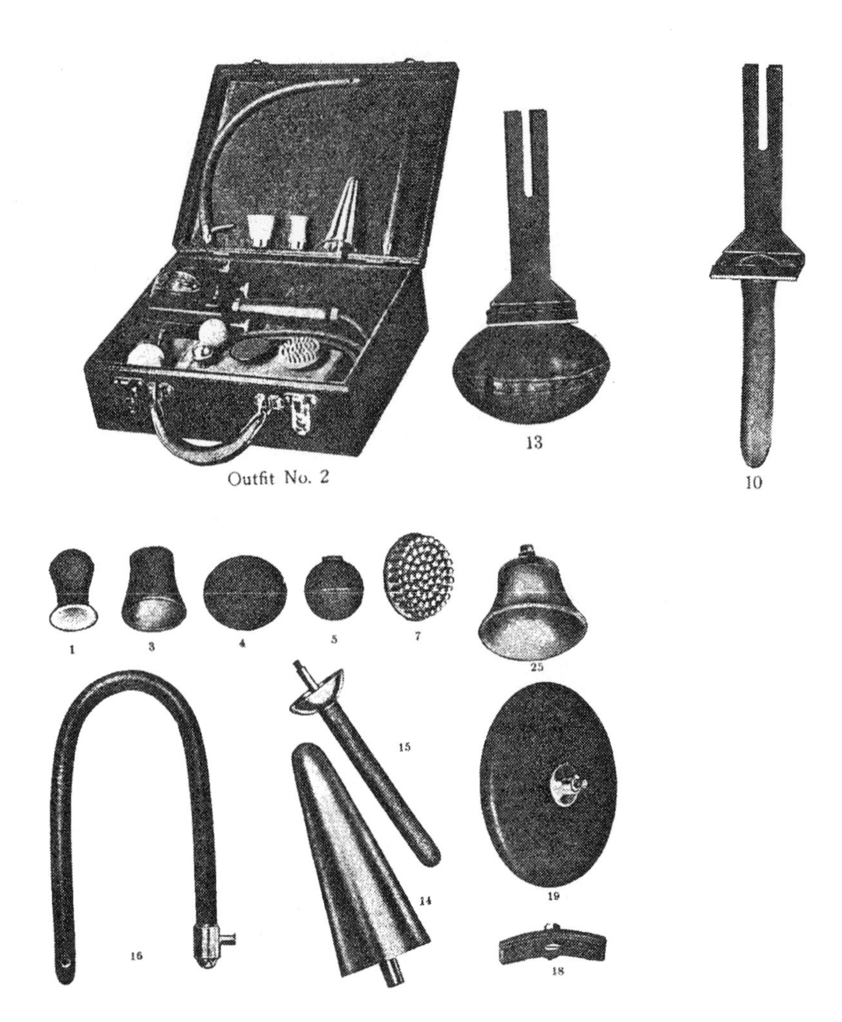

Fig. 21. Sam Gorman's "Physician's Vibragenitant," with set of vibratodes.

ical notions then popular in the medical community. D. T. Smith, for example, published a book in 1912 called *Vibration and Life*, which explained "Sex among Corpuscles" and the "Possibility of Race Betterment," among other topics related to the vibratory principles of the universe.[138] The vibrator's English godfather Mortimer Granville expounded on its theoretical underpinnings in rhetoric that was self-consciously scientific and rational:

> As a necessary result of this state of matters, it must be possible to act on the nervous system by purely mechanical agents and influences, with the effect of interrupting, modifying, or altogether arresting organic vibrations, whether in afferent sensory or efferent motor nerves. These effects are capable of demonstration, producing changes in the rate and rhythm of nerve vibration precisely correspondent with those which would be effected in the vibration of unorganized substances by the operation of the same or similar agents working in like processes.

Despite his disclaimer about percussing women, Mortimer Granville tells us that this theoretical understanding was arrived at "in connection with the paroxysmal, or recurrent, pains accompanying the uterine contractions in the natural process of parturition."[139]

Physicians clearly had an interest in maintaining their professional dignity, even as they sought methods of treating such "elusive" disorders as hysteria with therapies that would attract repeat business to their examining rooms. In some locations they faced competition with beauty parlors, which began using vibrators early in the twentieth century, "because the sensations from their use are pleasing and the results instanta-

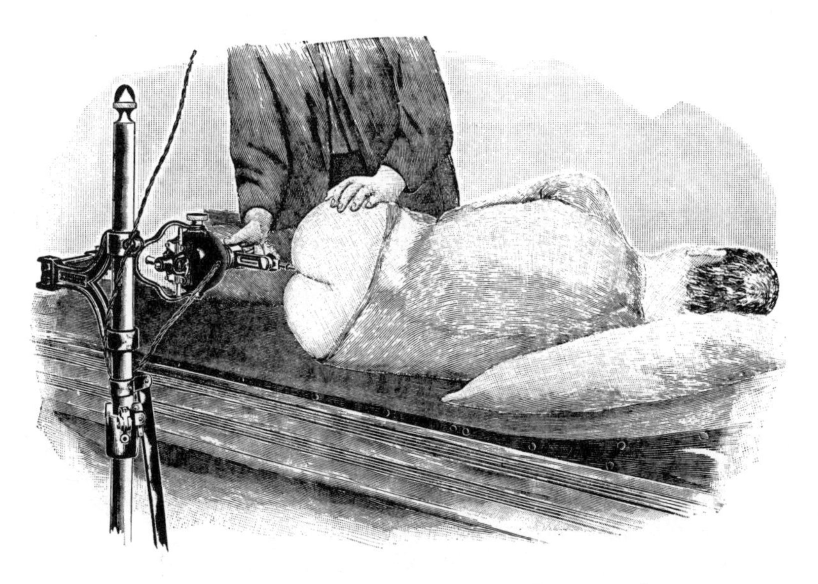

FIG. 22. The Chattanooga Vibrator in use on a male patient, about 1904.

neous."[140] Doctors were quite reasonably concerned, as a 1909 medical catalog expressed it, that "most of the vibrators sold by dealers and hawked about the country are mere trinkets which accomplish little more than titillation of the tissues."[141] Titillation of the tissues, however, had an attraction for some patients that there was no compelling reason to resist.

Consumer Purchase of Vibrators after 1900

A number of incentives made it more appealing for consumers to purchase vibrators for self-treatment at home than to visit a doctor's office regularly. The most obvious was cost: even a very good vibrator cost no more than four or five office visits, and it was available at all times, with no additional expenditure other than for electrical power. Consumers could use the device in privacy as often as they desired, and control it themselves, and the daring, knowledgeable, or shameless could involve their lovers or husbands. Water-powered vibrators, briefly popular in the first decades of this century, would have been poorly adapted to this purpose, but electromechanical devices, especially those with batteries, could be used anywhere. Increasing availability of home electricity must also have contributed to the popularity of the electromechanical vibrator.

The electrification of the home proceeded rapidly after the introduction of electric lights in 1876, and predictably, women were significant consumers of electrical appliances. The first home appliance to be electrified was the sewing machine in 1889, followed in the next ten years by the fan, the teakettle, the toaster, and the vibrator. The last preceded the electric vacuum cleaner by some nine years, the electric iron by ten, and the electric frying pan by more than a decade, possibly reflecting consumer priorities.[142] The earliest advertisement for a home vibrator I know of is for the "Vibratile," which appeared in *McClure's* in March 1899, offered as a cure for "Neuralgia, Headache, Wrinkles."[143] Much less sophisticated than medical models offered at the same period, the Vibratile had only one vibratode, a coil of wire.

Massage had been a subject of public interest since the days of Mesmer, and it lent itself to medical democratization at best and charlatanism at worst. Advertisements for home massage were common elements of the cornucopia of questionable products and services offered in popular publications in the early years of this century. The American College of Mechano-therapy, for example, announced to the readers of *Men and Women* in 1910, "Your Hands Properly Used are all You Need to Earn $3000 to $5000 a Year."[144] Mechanical massage devices operated by hand cranks advertised in this way included the Lambert Snyder, which, according to an advertisement in 1907, "Relieves All Suffering. Cures Disease." The device could "be placed in contact with any part of the body, and is capable of giving from 9,000 to 15,000 vibrations per minute." The Lambert Snyder sent "the red blood rushing into the congested parts, removing disease and pain."[145] The makers of the Bebout Vibrator, another hand-powered mechanical model, made their target market explicit in an ad in the *National Home Journal* in 1908: "TO WOMEN I address my message of health and beauty." The item sold by mail for $5 and was advertised in terms reminiscent of Wallian's alliterative rhapsodies on vibration in nature: "Gentle, soothing, invigorating and refreshing. Invented by a woman who knows a woman's needs. All nature pulsates and vibrates with life." Purchasers would find themselves in blissful harmony with the universe: "The most perfect woman is she whose blood pulses and oscillates in unison with the natural law of being."[146] Down the left column of the page on which the Bebout appears are small advertisements for "hair stain," nursing instruction by mail, furniture, broom clips, signet rings, ribbon, dropsy cures, postcards, poultry raising, matrimony, and rubber "Protectors" ("safe and sure, just the 'article' every woman wants"). Matchmaking was well represented, with three firms offering services, one of them offering "Pay when Married—New Plan."

At this period, not all urban water systems were metered. Water customers paid a flat rate to connect with the main, a practice that cities soon abandoned on discovering that consumers used water at a rate that overburdened wastewater disposal systems. There was no economic disincentive to using one's kitchen or bathroom faucet as a power source, and thus in the first two decades of the twentieth century there was a brief fashion for water-powered vibrators. On the embroidery page of

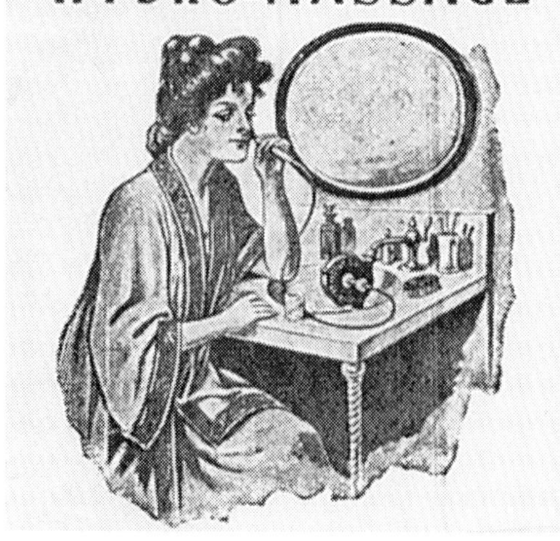

Fig. 23. The Warner Motor Company's water-powered "Hydro-massage," 1906.

the December 1906 issue of *Modern Women* the Warner Motor Company advertised a "Hydro-massage" machine operated from a kitchen or bathroom tap (fig. 23).[147] Amid ads for Palmolive soap, Onoto pens, cold cream, and lace, the May 1909 issue of *Woman's Home Companion* had a small display advertisement for the Corbin Vacuo-masseur, reportedly "Sold by Druggists and Department Stores," which apparently worked on hydraulic power as well.[148] The Blackstone Manufacturing Company offered a similar device ten years later; their ad in the April 1916 issue of *Hearst's* is aimed at attracting sales agents who want to "Get started in an honest, clean, reliable, money-making business."[149] Entrepreneurs who read *Hearst's* were evidently more economically upscale than subscribers to *Modern Women* and *Woman's Home Companion;* the other advertisements on the same page are for typewriters, law textbooks, a work on "The Power of Will," corn pads, and manufactured homes. The *Bohemian* of December 1909 advertised an electric massage roller resembling the "electro-spatteur" sold earlier as a medical instrument.[150]

The most numerous advertisements for vibrators in the first three decades of this century, however, were for electromechanical vibrators of the type that are still manufactured and sold for home massage. Popular magazines of the period accepted advertising for them but rarely mentioned them in editorial matter. Two exceptions are a one-liner in the June 1908 *Review of Reviews*, which cautions readers against "imprudence" and "excess in action" when using vibrators, and Mildred Maddocks's article about electricity in the July 1916 *Good Housekeeping*, in which her evaluation of vibrators is limited to the observation that they are "soothing to the skin."[151]

These soothing effects figured prominently in the advertising copy for vibrators and in the instruction manuals that accompanied them. The American Vibrator Company of St. Louis, Missouri, which advertised in *Woman's Home Companion* in 1906, stressed the superiority of its device over the unaided human hand:

> Why has electrical massage taken the place of the manual, or Swedish method? Simply because it can be applied more rapidly, uniformly and **deeply** than by hand, and for as long a period as may be desired. The professional masseur can not only not reach as deeply as can mechanical vibration, but is manifestly unable to prolong his treatment for a sufficient length of time to accomplish the results attained by modern vibratory machinery, which never tires. The number and strength of the movements that can be applied by hand are extremely limited; the perfectly adjusted American Vibrator runs **indefinitely** and is susceptible of a variety and rapidity of movements utterly impossible of human attainment. (Emphasis in the original)

Women were advised that the "American Vibrator may be attached to any electric light socket, **can be used by yourself** in the privacy of dressing room or boudoir, and furnishes every woman with the very essence of perpetual youth."[152] The Swedish Vibrator Company of Chicago sought sales agents for its product in the pages of *Modern Priscilla* of April 1913, extolling the device as "a machine that gives 30,000 thrilling, invigorating, penetrating, revitalizing vibrations per minute." A brief demonstration would be sure to win customers' approval, since they would have an "Irresistible desire to own it" after experiencing "the living, pulsing touch of its rhythmic vibratory motion." On the same page is an advertisement for Professor Burns's "Auto-Masseur . . . Both sexes," which was apparently a kind of corset.[153] The Monarch Vibrator Company had a small display ad in the February 1916 issue of *Hearst's Magazine*, showing a young woman pressing the cup vibratode to her right temple and claiming that their instrument would "bring SOCIAL AND BUSINESS SUCCESS . . . If your circulation is poor, its smooth, *passive exercise* sends the blood coursing through veins and tissues. Wrinkles disappear, hollows fill up, weariness ceases, and you learn the real joy of living."[154] In a contiguous advertisement, William Lee Howard's book *Sex Problems in Worry and Work* promises to answer questions such as, "Is Chastity Consistent with Health?" and to elucidate "The Sexual Problem of the Neurasthenic."[155] General Electric featured a vibrator in a full-page advertisement for "The Home Electrical" between 1915 and 1917.[156]

Mail order was a standard method of marketing vibrators between 1900 and 1920. The J. J. Duck Company of Toledo, Ohio, for example, offered a vibrator in its 1912 catalog *Anything Electrical* for $17.50, about $10 less than it charged for a five-car electric train.[157] Sears, Roebuck and Company published an *Electrical Goods* catalog in 1918 that emphasized the modernity and efficiency of electrical appliances for the home. Among these were coffee urns, toasters, irons, heaters, hair dryers, and other such devices, as well as home electromedical apparatus. Sears offered three kinds of home medical batteries at prices ranging from $4.95 to $11.95, three violet ray devices, and six models of vibrator, plus the vibratory attachment for a home motor described in chapter 1 (fig. 24). Vibrators ranged in price from a low of $5.95 to a deluxe "professional" model with numerous applicators and vibratodes at $28.75.[158] In the twenties and early thirties, some brands of vibrator, such as the Star, were available at retail; print advertising advised male readers to purchase the devices as gifts for women. In 1922 two models of Star vibrators, "Such Delightful Companions!" were available, a deluxe model at $12.50 and a portable that retailed for $5, with "six feet of cord. Comes in good-looking black box. Perfect for week-end trips."[159] Violet ray devices and apparatus combining violet rays with electromechanical vibration were available in 1932 in the United States, the United Kingdom, and Canada. According to their endorsers, "either Pulsation Massage or Suction Massage may be enjoyed," noting that the glass and rubber applicators may be used "with every comfort and safety on the delicate parts of the face and body."[160]

By far the most widely advertised home vibrator of the early twen-

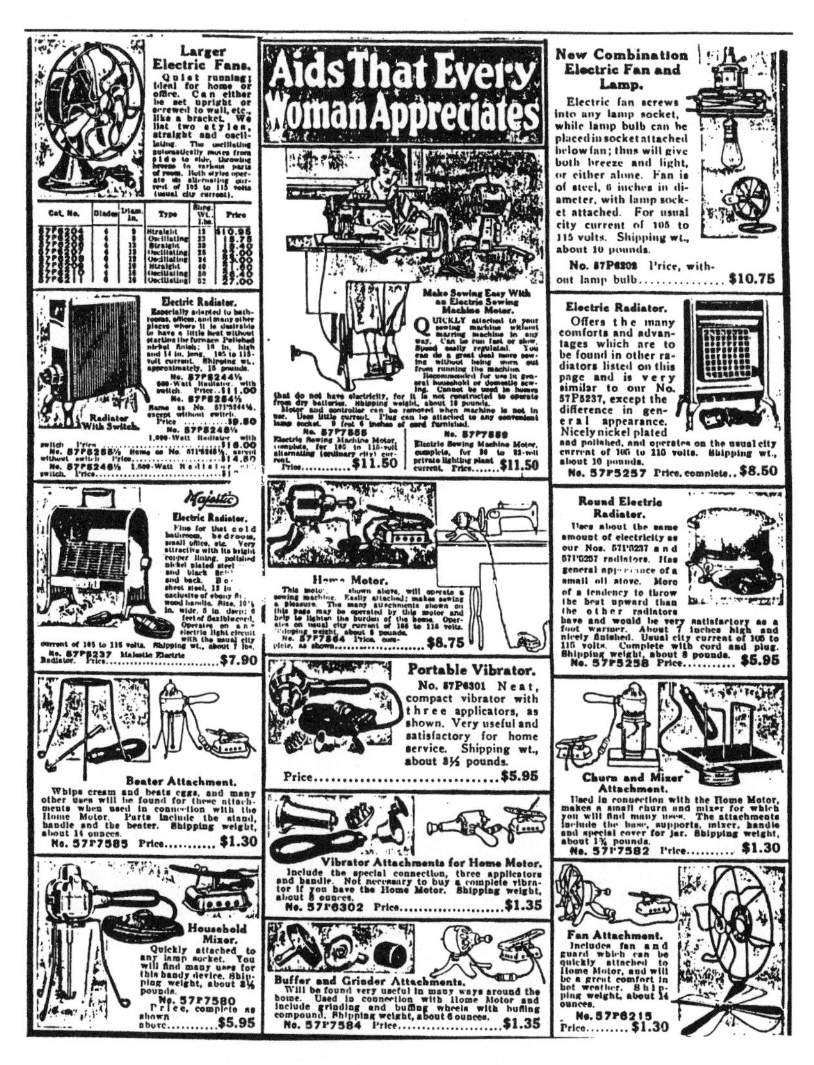

Fig. 24. "Aids That Every Woman Appreciates," Sears, Roebuck and Company, 1918.

tieth century, however, was that of the Lindstrom Smith Company of Chicago, whose White Cross Electric Vibrators (fig. 25) were sold from about 1902 through the 1930s as "Swedish Movement right in your own home." Advantages to purchasers included the savings over massage

Vibration is Life

The secret of the ages has been discovered in *Vibration*. Great scientists tell us that we owe not only our health but even our life strength to this wonderful force. Vibration promotes life and vigor, strength and beauty.

Vibration is one of the most marvelous curative agent known. It is the remedy provided by nature for many ills and diseases. It relieves like magic. Simple, easy and inexpensive—it banishes drugs forever.

Vibrate Your Body and Make It Well

YOU Have No Right to Be Sick!

Relieving Stomach Trouble With Vibration.

Pain, suffering and disease are unnatural—they are wrong. It is your **duty** to be well. Don't try to stand pain—STOP IT. No matter what ails you—even if others have told you that your case was incurable—DON'T GIVE UP HOPE. The great natural forces, **Vibration and Electricity**, are recognized to-day as among the greatest of curative agencies. The great

WHITE CROSS Electric Vibrator

combines **both** of these great natural curative agents. It gives you your choice of Vibration, Faradic and Galvanic Electricity, either separately or in combination, just as you wish. It relieves pain and its **effects are permanent.**

The White Cross Electric Vibrator gets at the **cause** of disease. It sends the rich, red blood leaping and coursing through your veins and arteries **straight to where the disease begins**, and where there is rich blood it is impossible for disease to remain long. It tones up your nerves and muscles and every vital organ. It makes you **fairly tingle with the joy of living.**

Don't neglect the FIRST symptoms. If you feel "run down," out of condition, if you feel "out of sorts" generally, **something is wrong.** The **most serious** diseases creep upon you unawares. **The White Cross Electric Vibrator** aids in filling our body so full of vigorous, robust health that pain and disease have a hard time finding a foothold.

Making the Hair Beautiful with Vibration

Vibration for the Racking Backache of Women.

READ WHAT OTHERS SAY

MAKES A VIBRATING CHAIR EQUAL TO CHAIRS SELLING FOR $180.00

Kansas City, Mo.

Lindstrom-Smith Co., Chicago, Ill.

Gentlemen:—The latter part of June or the first of July last I purchased of you the White Cross Electric Vibrator, and I will say that we have been very much pleased with it. My wife has had spinal trouble from a child and has been subject to severe headaches for a period of thirty-five years. The Vibrator has always relieved her headaches immediately, greatly helps her spinal trouble, and [illegible] from the very start. My wife says she would not part with the machine. We have used the vibrating chair by means of the chair attachment, and a friend [illegible] says it is equal to a vibrating chair that he used and cost $180.00. Very truly yours,

[illegible]

WOULD NOT TAKE $1,000 FOR IT

Los Angeles, Calif.

Lindstrom-Smith Co., Chicago, Ill.

Gentlemen:—I bought one of your No. 3 Vibrators last June and at that time I was a nervous wreck; was taking treatments a week from one of the best physicians in Los Angeles $2.00 for each treatment, and as they were helping me I thought it would be far cheaper to have the vibrator in my own home, hence my order. I received the machine on the 17th of June and began to take both the vibratory and electric treatments according to directions. To-day I can honestly say I am cured of my nervous trouble entirely. I am mentally and physically a stronger woman. My case was of 14 years' standing. Would not take $1,000.00 for my Vibrator if I could not get another like it. Very truly yours,

2007 [illegible] Street. C. B. FREER

PREFER IT TO MANY HIGH-PRICED MACHINES

Goshen, Okla.

Lindstrom-Smith Co., Chicago, Ill.

Gentlemen:—There is no other machine on the market for the same money as good and I prefer it to many higher priced ones for several practical reasons. Very respectfully,

Box 85. DR. SAM. L. WHITMORE

THE VIBRATING CHAIR IS FINE FOR THAT TIRED FEELING

Buffalo, N. Y.

Lindstrom-Smith Co., Chicago, Ill.

Gentlemen:—I would not take the price I gave for the vibrator if I could not get another. The benefit I have received for my eyesight and bronchial trouble is of great value. The Vibrating Chair is fine for that tired, exhausted feeling. As far as I have used the vibrator I can speak in favorable terms. Respectfully yours,

34 Rhode Island St. MRS. R. A. [illegible]

HELPED NASAL CATARRH AND WATERY EYES

Appleton, Wis.

Lindstrom-Smith Co., Chicago, Ill.

Gentlemen:—The vibrator came all right. I have used it for nasal catarrh and watery eyes and headaches and it has helped them. I believe it will be a good thing. Yours truly,

J. H. HOLDEMAN

CURES CONSTIPATION OF THREE YEARS' STANDING

Juneau

Lindstrom-Smith Co., Chicago, Ill.

Dear Sirs:—I have been using one of your No. 3 Vibrators for over a month. I find it very beneficial for the stomach and bowel trouble. It has cured me of Chronic Constipation of over three years standing. I am feeling fine. The Faradic power has done wonders for me in with the vibrator. The chair is surely a success. I would surely recommend it to anyone that is troubled with stomach trouble and constipation.

Juneau, Alaska. W. H. TOWNSEND

REMOVED WRINKLES

Cleveland, Ohio

Lindstrom-Smith Co., Chicago, Ill.

I have used the vibrator but two weeks and I find it removes wrinkles. Respectfully,

MRS. G. ROSE

CURES SCIATICA AND LUMBAGO

Rushsville, Okla.

Lindstrom-Smith Co., Chicago, Ill.

Dear Sirs:—We are much pleased with the machine, and I have already cured a friend of sciatica and lumbago. Yours truly,

MRS. GERTRUDE CLARK

HELPED HEADACHE

San Antonio, Texas

Lindstrom-Smith Co., Chicago, Ill., Box 572.

Gentlemen:—My vibrator has certainly helped my head. I have not had a spell of headache since getting it and that is nearly two months. Respectfully,

MRS. ANNA WUNDER

[illegible] St., Sta. A. San Antonio, Texas

Vibrating Chair FREE

With the White Cross Vibrator you can make a splendid vibrating chair out of any chair. A chair which will give you the same results as the kind used in the biggest hospitals and sanitariums. You cannot do this with any other vibrator in the world. **Swedish movement** right in your own home. You can give yourself the very same treatments for which specialists and sanitariums charge from $2.00 to $3.00 each. Nervous, irritable, worn-out men and women have obtained quicker and more permanent benefit from a few minutes each day in the vibrating chair than from hundreds of dollars worth of medicine. Send the free coupon attached to this announcement and let us explain all about our great special offer which we are making. Let us show you how you can make **any chair** a vibrating chair and without a cent of extra expense.

Enjoying the Tingling, Health-Giving Sensation of the Vibrating Chair

A Picture of the Wonderful White Cross Electric Vibrator,

The only vibrator in the world which combines the three great forces of Vibration, Galvanic and Faradic Electricity is shown here. This is the very same machine which has relieved hundreds of cases which had been given up as incurable. Read the letters printed on this page. These letters are from people who know what the White Cross Electric Vibrator is and what it can and does do. You should not delay. You should send the free coupon now—at once. You should get our free book, "Health and Beauty."

This Valuable Book, "Health and Beauty," Now Sent FREE

This wonderful book describes the human body in health and disease so plainly and clearly that anyone can understand. It tells how to get healthy and beautiful and how to keep so. This book tells you what vibration will do for you and how you can get the White Cross Electric Vibrator sent to you for an actual free trial. Whether you are sick or well you should send for this book anyway. You cannot tell when you may need it and need it badly. When you do there will be no time to send for it. Learn to-day what vibration will do for you—for all your loved ones. Learn all about its wonderful health-giving powers. Learn how you can save drug bills and treat yourself at home without expense. **Our Free Book** tells you how to relieve headache, catarrh, insomnia, backache, indigestion, rheumatism, neuralgia, earache, nervous debility, heart trouble, deafness, stomach trouble, scalp disease, constipation and lumbago: these and many other chronic and acute ailments all successfully treated by vibration. Get the **Free Book Now.**

HEALTH AND BEAUTY

Send This FREE Coupon

Don't Delay. Send this Free Coupon now. Clip out and mail at once so you have [illegible] without sending. You owe it to yourself to send this coupon to us and find out all about our

Great Special Limited Offer

For a short time only the price of our vibrators are greatly reduced on our tremendous introductory offer. Write to-day for the great special offer and our **Free Book, "Health and Beauty."** Send the coupon. No letter is necessary—the coupon will do—but send at once.

LINDSTROM-SMITH CO.

253 La Salle St., Dept. 1899

CHICAGO, ILL.

SIGN THIS COUPON AND MAIL TO-DAY

Lindstrom-Smith Co., 253 La Salle St., Dept. 1899, Chicago, Ill.

Without obligations on me please send me free your special reduced price offer, free book on Health and Beauty, treatment of disease by vibration and electricity, and complete catalog.

Name..........

Address..........

Write plainly

FIG. 25. "Vibration is Life," advertisement for Lindstrom Smith's White Cross Vibrator, from *Modern Priscilla*, 1910.

treatments in a doctor's office and the privacy of self-treatment at home.[161] The brand, White Cross, was drawn from the name of an Episcopalian sexual purity organization that flourished in Britain in the late 1880s. The society was introduced to America by Frances Willard of the Women's Christian Temperance Union; its name on the Lindstrom Smith vibrator must have been intended to suggest virtue and chastity.[162] Advertisements in *Needlecraft*, *Home Needlework Magazine*, *American Magazine*, *Modern Priscilla*, the *National Home Journal*, and *Hearst's* between 1908 and 1916 told women:

> You can relieve pain, stiffness and weakness, and you can make the body plump and build it up with thrilling, refreshing vibration and electricity. Just a few minutes' use of the wonderful vibrator and the red blood tingles through your veins and arteries and you feel vigorous, strong and well. With our Electric Vibrator and special attachments you can convert **any chair** into a perfect vibrating chair without extra cost, getting the genuine Swedish Movement and wonderfully refreshing effects, the same treatment for which you would have to pay at least $2.00 each in a physician's office.[163]

Sharing a page with the White Cross in the *National Home Journal* is an advertisement for Wade's Golden Nervine for "Weak Men." In the December 1910 *Modern Priscilla*, a woman is shown vibrating her coccyx and a man his stomach; the copy claims that their product eliminates the causes of disease by sending "the rich, red blood leaping and coursing through your veins and arteries," which in turn "makes you fairly tingle with the joy of living." A somewhat alarming testimonial claims that the White Cross "Cured Constipation of Three Years' Standing."[164] The *American Magazine* of January 1913 had an advertisement for the White Cross showing a young woman in suggestive dishabille, applying the ball vibratode to the upper surface of her right breast. Enthusiastic boldface and italics punctuate the text:

> Rests, strengthens, renews, repairs. Every vital organ is *crammed full of vitality*. The clogging waste is *swept away* by the coursing blood which the marvelous force sets leaping through every vein and artery *with the virile strength of perfect health*. You sleep as restfully **as you used to.** You awaken, *refreshed* mentally—physically—*strong in mind and body* and **glad to be alive.**[165]

A later advertisement in the same magazine included the orgasmic phraseology quoted in chapter 1:

> Vibration is life. It will chase away the years like magic. Every nerve, every fibre of your whole body will tingle with force of your own awakened powers. All the keen relish, the pleasures of youth, will throb within you. **Rich, red blood** will be sent coursing through your veins and you will realize thoroughly the joy of living. Your self-respect, even, will be increased a hundredfold.[166]

The December 1928 advertising section of *Popular Mechanics* included a half-page ad for Lindstrom and Company's "Elco Electric Health Generator," a vibrator with violet ray and ozone capacity apparently marketed to families rather than explicitly to women as in the earlier advertisements.[167] Vibrator advertising then disappeared from home magazines until the modern vibrator resurfaced in the 1960s as a frankly sexual toy.[168]

In the 1950s, massager (but not vibrator) advertisements did appear in some downmarket magazines for women, such as *Workbasket*, an inexpensive needlework periodical printed on pulp paper from 1930 through the mid-1960s. Called "Spot Reducers," "Glorifier Massagers" ("Take Off Ugly Fat"), or "Massage Pillows," these devices had flat working surfaces and no attachments or vibratodes, although one, the Viber-8, could be fastened under the chin. Many of the advertisements, however, conspicuously feature applications to the abdomen.[169]

Roger Blake, admittedly not the most reliable of historians, calls vibrators the "oldest sex gadget of the twentieth century" and mentions the appearance of the vibrator in erotic films in the 1920s. He describes a movie called "Widow's Delight" in which "a finely dressed matron" rejects a kiss at the door from her well-dressed male escort, "then dashes into her bedroom and within seconds is stripped to her open girdle and stockings. She produces one of the first vibrator models on the market, with the motor largely exposed, and applies it liberally to her privates."[170] It seems likely that this kind of exposure helped to drive the vibrator from the medical and respectable home markets, since it made social camouflage very difficult to maintain.

Other factors must have contributed as well, such as the growing understanding by both men and women of female sexual function, making it difficult to disguise the use of vibrators by either physicians or consumers as a mere therapeutic measure. Decades later, when the vibrator reemerged in advertising from its midcentury eclipse, few efforts were made to camouflage its sexual benefits.

Vibrators may not have been advertised in respectable publications, at least in the United States between about 1930 and the 1970s, but they must have been available. Albert Ellis does not seem to think, in 1963, that his readers will require any explanation of the assertion that one of the many techniques of arousing women to orgasm is "massage of their external genitalia with electric vibrators."[171] Paul Tabori, as well, expects in 1969 that Americans will be familiar with the use of both vibrators and massagers as "marital aids."[172] The chief difficulties of the device in the latter half of the twentieth century seem to have been male dismay at its efficacy compared with their own efforts and female ambivalence about the possibility of "addiction" to the multiple orgasms the device so effortlessly produced.[173] Helen Singer Kaplan wrote in 1974, "The vibrator provides the strongest, most intense stimulation known. Indeed, it has been said that the electric vibrator represents the only significant advance in sexual technique since the days of Pompeii."[174] Even sex therapists, who conceded that the vibrator was an effective treatment for some kinds of sexual "dysfunction," were slow to endorse it for "normal" heterosexual relations.[175] Edward Dengrove, who had great hopes in 1971 for the vibrator as a sex aid, observed that some women did not want to use vibrators because they believed that only vaginal orgasms were desirable, and that "men are likely to reject its use because it makes them out to be incapable of producing orgasm in the female on their own; emasculating them, so to speak."[176]

Some feminists have expressed highly ambivalent opinions of the vibrator. In Susan Strasser's 1982 history of housework, *Never Done*, the author and one of her sources revile the invention, along with other modern expressions of female sexuality, in almost puritanical terms:

> Sexual massage parlors and public pornography appeal primarily to men; despite *Playgirl* and bars with male go-go dancers, most women prefer to keep sex private, and many have bought themselves machines for sex partners. The vibrator—a one-time purchase that requires even less conversa-

tion than a prostitute—has left the sex shops and now appears in department and variety stores, manufactured by the same respectable corporations that market electric razors and hair dryers, with names like Feelin' Good and Body Language, and instruction booklets that refer to a "soft touch body massager for . . . tender areas." Sex researchers and therapists agree that the vibrator's intense stimulation produces orgasms fast and consistently; many recommend them to patients, sometimes with warnings about the possibility of dependence on the gadget. The housewares industry's entry to the market takes the device beyond therapy; as one writer points out, it "poses new questions: has achieving orgasm become just another way of releasing the tensions of day-to-day living? Has the vibrator, once considered a therapeutic device, become a sort of microwave oven of the bedroom—a fast, efficient means of getting sexual pleasure? Is the most efficient orgasm the best orgasm? Is the bedroom really the place for a time-saving device? If so, what are we saving all this time for?"[177]

Both Strasser and the author she quotes seem unaware that the "respectable" housewares industry has been involved in the production and sale of vibrators for nearly a century, and they fail to note that women have traditionally lacked the methods of "releasing the tensions of day-to-day living" available to men.

But a persistent theme in the background of these concerns about the vibrator is the classic male fear of sexual inadequacy, to which the new technology adds a threat once associated only with industrial artisans: technological obsolescence.

5

Revising the Andro-centric Model

Orgasmic Treatment in the Practice of Western Medicine

The history of physical therapies for hysteroneurasthenic disorders as I have discussed it here tells us several things about Western physicians. Some we already knew. For example, that normal conditions can be medicalized, especially in women, has been widely observed concerning masturbation, pregnancy, and menstruation. That doctors both create and become invested in dominant social and medical paradigms is also well known; Haller, Foucault, and Gay have all directed our attention to physicians' roles as arbiters and recorders of sexual behavior. That disease paradigms go in and out of fashion has been widely noted, by Brumberg, Shorter, Figlio, Hudson, and many others. I have already mentioned some of the feminist sources on hysteria, which highlight its character as a feminine pathology even in men.

Mirko Grmek and others have pointed out that history's physicians have had to deal with a bewildering universe. They have been frustrated by the organic complexity of the living body and its opacity to scientific observation, hampered by inadequate instrumentation and testing techniques. Added to the awe-inspiring biochemical and physiological mysteries of the human organism have been mental processes and behaviors, which often defy efforts to arrange them neatly within the framework of scientific theory. We should hardly be surprised that sexuality, existing at the intersection of the mind and the body and bearing heavy, sometimes impenetrable overlays of social construction, should have been subject to successive waves of medical interpretation.

What is impressive, however, is that the androcentric paradigm of sexuality—that sex consists of penetration (usually of the vagina) to male orgasm—is a fixed point in the otherwise shifting sands of Western medical opinion. By 1930 Freud's notion that women had two types of orgasms, clitoral and vaginal, of which only the latter was mature and healthy, had become the dominant paradigm of normative female sexuality. It was to persist well into the 1970s. Galenism and Freudianism had few points of agreement, but they concurred that orgasm for both parties during heterosexual coitus was the healthiest form of sexual expression. Clearly the cultural emphasis on intercourse is so deeply entrenched that physicians simply do not perceive it in themselves and their patients. And what they do not notice, they cannot question. Certainly there is an understandably pro-natal bias in Western medical practice, beginning with Hippocrates, but there is more to it than that. There is a systematic effort to subsume the knowledge that the clitoris, not the vagina, is the seat of greatest sexual feeling in most women into the androcentric model and to avoid one-to-one heterosexual confrontation over orgasmic mutuality by shifting the dispute onto medical ground.

When physicians from John Pechey to David Reuben have instructed men to stimulate the clitoris, this advice has been given mainly in the context of a prelude or adjunct to coitus. There typically is great concern that the male partner not be significantly inconvenienced. To take a modern example, Alexander Lowen, writing of his medical experiences with female sexuality in 1965, did not like to recommend clitoral stimulation to his patients because "most men . . . feel that the need to bring a woman to climax through clitoral stimulation is a burden." If coitus is delayed while the man brings the woman to orgasm in this way, "it imposes a restraint upon his natural desire for closeness and intimacy," possibly resulting in a loss of his erection, and "the subsequent act of coitus is deprived of its mutual quality." During coitus, he may employ clitoral stimulation to "help the woman to reach a climax, but it distracts the man from the perception of his genital sensations and greatly interferes with the pelvic movements upon which his own feeling of satisfaction depends." Bringing his partner to orgasm after his own climax will not do either, "since it prevents him from enjoying the relaxation and peace that are the rewards of sexuality. Most men to whom I have spoken who engaged in this practice resented it."[1]

Lowen shows here what Sophie Lazarsfeld calls "the cloven hoof of the true masculine view."[2] In this text it is quite clear that women who need clitoral stimulation to reach orgasm are thought to be making unfair and unreasonable demands on their male partners, and that life would be simpler for all concerned if they would simply adjust to the androcentric model and have their orgasms vaginally. Lowen wrote at a time when it was no longer possible to simply hand off the job of producing orgasm to a physician or midwife. When the one-to-one confrontation cannot be avoided, Lowen expects the woman to yield.

This raises another question about orgasmic treatment as a medical procedure: its parallels with prostitution. There have been many arguments, historical and modern, regarding whether it should be legal for women and men to sell the service of producing orgasm. Some feminists in this and previous centuries have argued that there cannot be prostitution without systematic degradation of its practitioners.[3] In the case of Western physicians, the legal question apparently never arose, although, as we have seen, there was some controversy within the profession as to the propriety of vulvular massage. Physicians, unlike prostitutes, did not lose status by providing sexual services, in part because the character of these services was camouflaged both by the disease paradigms constructed around female sexuality and by the comforting belief that only penetration was sexually stimulating to women. Thus the speculum and the tampon were originally more controversial in medical circles than was the vibrator. The aura of respectability that physicians cast over their provision of sexual services suggests that the task of producing orgasm is not in itself demeaning; performing it did not cause loss of caste for its elite practitioners, who were capable of disguising its earthy character.

As I observed earlier, there is no evidence that physicians as a class enjoyed performing these services for their patients, apart from the not unrelated satisfactions of providing needed therapy and collecting their fees. Some, perhaps, may have taken more intimate liberties, but we have no evidence that such behaviors were widespread. On the contrary, when technology or midwife assistants could get the job done, doctors seem to have been more than willing to lighten the burden of massage therapies. Physicians seem to have been no more eager to take on the task of producing orgasm in women than were the sexual partners who sent them for therapy, but the doctors were paid for their services. Moreover, since physicians for the most part seem to have regarded these therapies simply as routine clinical tasks, the necessity for such stimulation did not interfere with their own sexual enjoyment, as it reportedly did with male sexual partners.

Doctors who employed physical therapies for hysteria and related female disorders wanted the means of providing them to be routine, convenient, and affordable. Since physicians at all times and places have had to acquire a large number of very diverse skills, any area of practice that could be partially deskilled by instruments represented an advance in efficiency not only of practice but also of education. As Nathaniel Highmore tells us, vulvular massage was difficult to learn, an obstacle removed by the invention of the vibrator in the nineteenth century. Hysterical patients must have been a good source of cash flow, since they were in no mortal danger from their illness and required regular treatment.

Finally, it must be conceded that the therapy is by no means inappropriate to many of the manifestations of what was known until 1952 as a disease: orgasm usually does relieve such symptoms as pelvic hyperemia, sleeplessness, anxiety, headaches, and nervousness. At the very worst, the physicians in question have been true to the Hippocratic injunction to do no harm.

The Androcentric Model in Heterosexual Relationships

We have seen that the hysteroneurasthenic disorders have been the focus of an elaborate network of controversies over the past two and a half millennia. Since 1952 their definition has been so substantially altered as to rule out many of the clinical descriptions of history. This, of course, is not unusual in medicine: physicians no longer diagnose their patients as plethoric or choleric, and "died of a fever" would be considered unacceptably imprecise on a modern death certificate. Historically, there has been controversy over whether hysteria was necessarily a female disease, but it was clear when Charles Mills wrote of it in 1886 that only a minority of physicians believed men could have the disorder and that even they were convinced that only a very few hysterics were male.[4] Most of the debates among clinicians have been over proper methods of treatment, including the production of orgasm. If marriage and intercourse failed to cure hysterical women, some doctors, at least, were convinced that responsibility for producing the necessary therapeutic effect rested with them. It is interesting that though marriage and intercourse were sometimes recommended for hysterical males, I have found no accounts of therapeutic massage of the male genitalia by physicians.

Many questions can and should be raised about the persistence of Western belief that women ought to reach orgasm during heterosexual coitus. Certainly, its importance to impregnation must have contributed to our doggedly maintaining it in the face of abundant individual and societal evidence that penetration unaccompanied by direct stimulation of the clitoris is an inefficient and, more often than not, ineffective way to produce orgasm in women.[5] It is hardly worth belaboring the point that most men enjoy coitus and that men have been the dominant sex through most of Western history. Yet the fact remains of our normative preference for coitus, in which the constant from Hippocrates to Freud—despite breathtaking changes in nearly every other area of medical thought—is that women who do not reach orgasm by means of penetration alone are sick or defective. The penetration myth is not a conspiracy perpetuated by men; women too want to believe in the ideal of universal orgasmic mutuality in coitus. Even the sexual radical Wilhelm Reich could not see beyond this time-honored norm.[6] The feminist questioning of androcentric sexuality over the past three decades is recent and, one might say, long overdue.[7] Carole Vance, reporting on a 1977 "Program on Human Sexuality" conducted by the Center for Sex Research and funded by the National Institute of Mental Health, noted that in presentations at the program it was assumed that "all heterosexual contact culminated in vaginal penetration, indicating a progression through hierarchies of sexual activity, from the now acceptable normal 'foreplay' to 'real sex.' Heterosexual sex, then, requires genital contact, male erection, and penetration."

Vance goes on to describe one of the presentations, in which a psychiatrist recounted work with couples who reported "the female's inability to experience orgasm during vaginal penetration, although many of these women were orgasmic during masturbation or other forms of clitoral stimulation." When asked whether this state of affairs should, in fact, be considered a dysfunction requiring treatment, the psychiatrist replied that it should, whereas the opposite condition, ability to reach orgasm through penetration but not through masturbation, did not require therapeutic intervention.[8]

The personal and social cost to individual men and women of defying or questioning the androcentric model remains high enough to deter rebellion. Even historians, who are notoriously gimlet-eyed about cultural myths, have been reluctant to challenge the hypothesis that penetration of the vagina to male orgasm is the only kind of sex that matters and the only kind that can and should result in sexual bliss for women. Seymour Fisher observed in 1973 that "it is particularly remarkable how widespread has been the acceptance of assumptions about the 'more mature' nature of vaginal arousal in the absence of any empirical evidence to support them" and went on to say that 64 percent of his sample of women respondents preferred clitoral to vaginal stimulation.[9] The lack of correspondence between the observed data and the androcentric model, and the reasons the model persisted even among professionals, was analyzed by Jeanne Warner in 1984, in a discussion about the advantages of "emotional," rather than physical, orgasm for women. She argues for "a male bias for phallic stimulation" even though "the literature conveys a strong impression that the penis is not the most effective means of producing a maximal level of arousal and response for a woman." Arguments that "emotional orgasm" is superior to the physical kind "seem to suggest that whatever provides the greatest satisfaction for the male should also provide the greatest pleasure for the female."[10]

What is surprising about the androcentric hypothesis is not that it exists, which, as we have seen, is readily explained, but that we have been willing to sacrifice so much to it. Female orgasm is not necessary to conception, so it can take place (or not) outside the context of intercourse without interfering either with male enjoyment of sex or with conception. The central position in history occupied by these two concerns to a large extent explains the omissions, silences, and learned misunderstandings about female sexuality. As long as female orgasm could be medicalized, it did not have to be discussed, which would have called uncomfortable attention to its apparent conflict with the norm of coitus. Cultures such as existed in some parts of Asia, in which female orgasm was more smoothly integrated with patriarchy, at least encouraged married couples to explore methods and positions conducive to women's pleasure.

In our own culture there have been, and remain, powerful means of negatively reinforcing women's demands for orgasmic mutuality. A woman's admitting that coitus does not by itself ring her chimes is in some quarters still a confession of defect. In addition, Western men are expected to be born knowing how to satisfy women in much the same way as women are assumed to be born knowing how to cook. Men have in the past even been held responsible for women's sexuality; Frank Caprio told young husbands in 1952 that "the sexual awakening of the wife [was their] responsibility."[11] In light of these impossible standards, men have not traditionally been interested in truthful (and perhaps unflattering) answers to their questions about female satisfaction; even where such answers have been provided, a man has had the option of blaming the woman for her (and thus his) failure.[12] Medical advice writers like Caprio have traditionally provided such encouragement as the assertion that women's "fixation of the sexual instinct" on the clitoris is the result of "excessive manipulation." Most of the rest of Caprio's book is about the problem of female "frigidity" caused by such pathological "fixations."[13] Few women are prepared to expose their intimate behavior to this kind of socially supported criticism. For most women struggling with more pressing problems of economic survival and family harmony, the cost of fighting the androcentric norm would almost certainly have seemed greater than the very slender possibility of ultimate reward.[14]

In 1848 the French author Auguste Debay wrote that women should fake orgasm because "man likes to have his happiness shared."[15] He was neither the first nor the last to take this position. Celia Roberts and her coauthors, studying the faking of orgasm in a sample of college women, found that "in almost every woman's interview these practices were mentioned as something they did, at least some of the time." Male interviewees were nearly all certain that no woman had ever faked orgasm with them, an observation about which the authors remark, "Clearly, the refined performances which women are giving are extremely convincing." Female subjects explained their behavior by referring to a greater interest in preserving the stability of their relationships than in reaching orgasm on every occasion of intercourse.[16]

Despite the systematic perpetuation of ignorance and misunderstanding—by women as well as men—most heterosexual men have looked to the female orgasm to reinforce their self-respect as sexual beings. Michael Segell says that "according to one study, one of the four utilitarian aspects of the female orgasm is the boost it gives men's egos."[17] A thirty-three-year-old male interviewed by *Glamour* advised his fellows, "When you find a woman who can come to orgasm through penetration and not just clitoral stimulation, keep her. She's a rare and wondrous thing."[18] Clearly, for this man no other female characteristics matter. Inevitably, such pressures could push women in only one direction: toward pretending to reach orgasm when it did not occur.[19] The readers of *Mademoiselle* reported in the early 1990s that 69 percent of them had faked orgasm at least once.[20] Carol Tavris and Susan Sadd, reporting the results of a survey in 1977, include two quotations from their respondents:

> I have conducted my own little survey and I do not have one friend or acquaintance who has ever had a "real" orgasm through intercourse—only through clitoral stimulation. However, try convincing a *man* you don't have orgasms his way. He won't believe you. But challenging him that way can get quite interesting! I have never had an orgasm during sexual intercourse. To have an orgasm, I must have cunnilingus or manual clitoral stimulation. I know of women today who are faking orgasm during intercourse because they are too embarrassed to tell their husbands or lovers that no matter how long they keep their erection, they just can't make her have orgasm.[21]

Robert Francoeur says of orgasmic pressures on women in heterosexual relationships that "women are much more likely to pretend to have had an orgasm when they haven't" and points out that such pretense often results in "real problems of resentment and even anger with the partner."[22]

Not all women agree. Stephanie Alexander, writing in *Cosmopolitan* in 1995, asserts that faking orgasm is "just a matter of expediency, not to mention common courtesy." Regarding the cost of trying to explain why one has not reached orgasm, she asks, "When you have to get up for work the next morning, who has two spare hours to make him feel better about not making you feel great?"[23] In effect, these accounts suggest that half of the heterosexual couple is expected to sacrifice orgasmic mutuality in order to avoid the inevitable stresses on the relationship caused by rocking the androcentric boat. As a culture, we must value the androcentric norm very highly even to suggest that maintaining it is worth such a price.

In the second half of this century, the work of Masters and Johnson and their followers has made yet another sacrifice to the androcentric model of sexuality: the objectivity of scientific thinking. When these researchers chose their sample, they selected only women who regularly reached orgasm in coitus—an error, it is worth noting, not made by their predecessor Alfred Kinsey. That these women were a minority was already known at the time Masters and Johnson made their study, but it had apparently been decided that these outliers represented normality. It is generally held to be a principle of the scientific use of statistics that the experience of the majority represents the norm; that is, the normal range is the part of the curve directly under the bell on a line graph. Were it not for the very strong and apparently widespread bias in the direction of the androcentric norm, Masters and Johnson would have been the laughingstock of the medical community. This did not occur. Not until Shere Hite attacked the Masters and Johnson results in 1976 did questions begin to be raised about their methods of selection and interpretation. Errors of this kind not only have prevented us from understanding female orgasm as a physiological phenomenon but have diverted us from fully recognizing how individual and idiosyncratic sexual pleasure is for both sexes.

The reactions (and overreactions) to Hite's own study also reveal much about how vigorously we have been willing to defend the androcentric model. Her work was severely criticized on the grounds that participants were self-selected, a problem that had arisen not only with the Kinsey and the Masters and Johnson samples but with nearly every other survey of sexual practices in this country in the past hundred years. As a

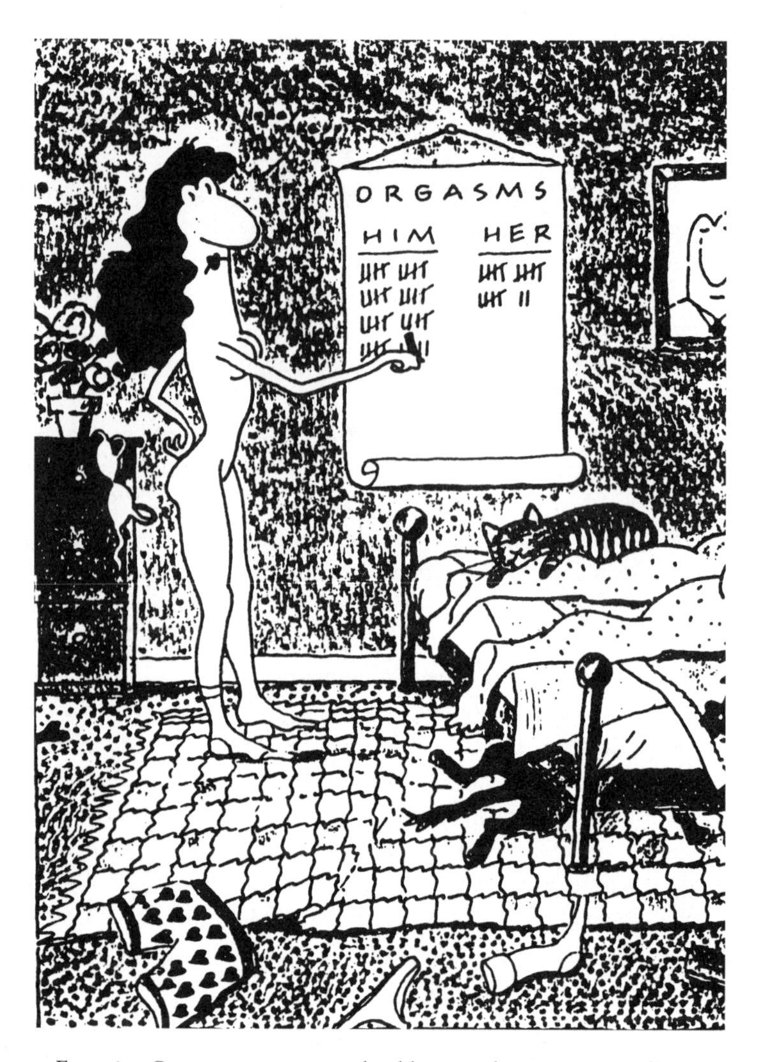

Fig. 26. Cartoon representing the dilemma of orgasmic mutuality in heterosexual relationships. The caption reads, "Wake up—honey . . . I think we need to have a talk." By Elizabeth W. Stanley and J. Blumner for the Maine Line Company, ca. 1986.

purely practical matter, people cannot be compelled to respond honestly to questions about intimate behavior; researchers have no choice but to rely on data whose representativeness is and must remain in doubt. In Hite's case, however, there were far more attempts to make this difficulty a fatal flaw than were made concerning her predecessors' work. Excuses of the most flimsy and embarrassingly male-centered kind were offered for rejecting Hite's hypothesis outright. In 1986, for example, the Hite reports were the subject of a session on the history of sexuality by the Organization of American Historians. One of the male participants criticized Hite's attention to the issue of orgasm in heterosexual relationships as "somewhat mechanistic." This is a very glib criticism from the side of such relationships that is having most of the orgasms.[24]

The Vibrator as Technology and Totem

As we have seen, the medicalizing of female orgasm in Western culture has been one means of protecting our comfortable illusions about coitus. The vibrator and its predecessor technologies—particularly manual and hydriatic massage—made it easy for physicians to provide the relief that was not otherwise accessible to many women. The vibrator was convenient, portable, and fast and thus enjoyed a considerable, if brief, popularity as a medical instrument before its discovery by consumers and by the makers of erotic films. The ultimate difficulty of the vibrator, from the point of view of the medical profession, was that it was so convenient and easy to use that it rendered unnecessary any medical intervention in the process of producing female orgasm. Hydriatic equipment and expensive office vibrators like the Chattanooga at least kept massage innovation in the hands of medical professionals; once the vibrator became a relatively lightweight and inexpensive device that could be operated by water or electricity in the home, it became a "personal care appliance" and not a medical instrument.

In the second half of this century the vibrator has become an overtly sexual device. Interestingly, when such devices appear in erotic films, it is rarely the true vibrator that is portrayed; what is seen is the reassuringly phallus-shaped vibrating dildo, with its suggestion that the machine is really only a substitute for a penis.[25] Edward Kelly, writing of vibrating dildos in 1974, avers hopefully that "without doubt, except in cases of lesbianism, the haunting vision of some imagined male broods over each use of any dildo."[26] For most women, however, these under-powered battery-operated toys are more visually than physiologically stimulating; it is the AC-powered vibrator with at least one working surface at a right angle to the handle that is best designed for application to the clitoral area.

Beyond the functional role of the vibrator for women consumers and their sexual partners, the device has taken on a totemic quality in American culture. Some male authors have pointed out that the vibrator makes an excellent addition to a couple's armamentarium of sex toys because it produces orgasm in women (and some men) with very little effort or skill. It has also become a favorite of sex therapists for the same reason—even women with very high orgasmic thresholds will usually respond eventually to vibratory massage. Those with lower thresholds can use the machine to explore their full orgasmic potential with very little fatigue. These two aspects of the vibrator have almost inevitably made it a focus of the kind of male fears played on by such jokes as, "When did God make men? When she realized that vibrators couldn't dance."[27] Since the Industrial Revolution, as Michael Adas has pointed out, men have tended to measure themselves against machines, a comparison virtually guaranteed to produce anxiety.[28] In the case of vibrators, this tension is especially poignant and has sometimes led men to resent the device. As one of the *Redbook* survey's respondents said of her adventures with her vibrator, "My husband doesn't know. If he did, I think he'd throw it out!"[29]

The late Melvin Kranzberg has been widely quoted in the observation that "technology is neither good nor bad; nor is it neutral."[30] The vibrator and its predecessors, like all technologies, tell us much about the societies that produced and used them. The device remains with us, praised by some and reviled by others, neither good, bad, nor neutral, a controversial focus of debate about female sexuality. Some of this controversy, as we have seen, has very old roots in Western culture, occupying the space in which sexuality, morality, and medicine interact and serving as an outer line of defense of the androcentric model of orgasmic mutuality in coitus. The rifts in this ancient wall continue to be patched with exhortations to women to avoid challenging the norm even if it means faking orgasm and sacrificing honesty in their intimate relationships with men. In the past we have been willing to pay this price; whether we should continue to do so is a question for individuals, not historians, to decide.

Notes

Preface

1. This, of course, was to some extent a misperception on my part. Actually, several people were doing it. See, for example, Susan Burroughs Swan, *Plain and Fancy* (New York: Holt, Rinehart and Winston, 1977); Florence Peto, *Historic Quilts* (New York: American Historical Company, 1939); Patsy Orlofsky and Myron Orlofsky, *Quilts in America* (New York: McGraw-Hill, 1974); Cuesta Benberry, articles in *Quilters' Newsletter* and *Nimble Needle Treasures* (1972–76); and Patricia Mainardi, "Quilts: The Great American Art," *Feminist Art Journal*, winter 1973, among others. There were a few sources on embroidery and the bobbin and needle-made laces, but there was virtually no secondary literature on hand knitting, crochet, and tatting.

2. Rachel Maines, "American Needlework in Transition, 1880–1930," *University of Michigan Papers in Women Studies*, 1978, 57–84.

3. "Grant Received," *Summer Bulletin*, Clarkson University (Potsdam, N.Y.), July 1, 1985, 5.

4. My husband refers to this IEEE episode as the Attack of the Dweebs.

Chapter 1 The Job Nobody Wanted

1. Alemarianus Petrus Forestus [Pieter van Foreest], *Observationem et Curationem Medicinalium ac Chirurgicarum Opera Omnia* (Rouen: Bertherlin, 1653), vol. 3, bk. 28.

2. A. E. Hanson, "Hippocrates: Diseases of Women," *Signs* 1, no. 2 (1975): 567–84; Aretaeus Cappadox, "On the Causes and Symptoms of Acute Diseases,"

in *The Extant Works of Aretaeus the Cappadocian*, ed. and trans. Francis Adams (London: Sydenham Society, 1856), bk. 2, chap. 2; Aulus Cornelius Celsus, *On Medicine*, trans. W. G. Spencer (Cambridge: Harvard University Press, 1935), vol. 1, chap. 4; Galen of Pergamon, *De Locis Affectis*, trans. Rudolf Siegel (New York: S. Karger, 1976), sec. 39; Soranus of Ephesus, *Gynecology*, trans. Owsei Temkin (Baltimore: Johns Hopkins Press, 1956), chap. 4; Äetius of Amida, "Tetrabiblion," bk. 16, chap. 67, trans. James Ricci, in *The Gynaecology and Obstetrics of the Sixth Century A.D.* (Philadelphia: Blakiston, 1950); Mustio, *La "Gynaecia" de Muscione*, ed. and trans. Rino Radicchio (Pisa: Giardini, 1970), 122; Rhazes, *Opus Medicinae Practicae Saluberrimum antehoc Nusquam Impressum, Galeatij de Sancta Sophia in Nonum Tractatum Libri Rhasis ad Regem Almansorum* (Hagenou: Valentini Kobian, 1533); Avicenna, *Liber de Anima, seu Sextus de Naturalibus* (Leiden: Brill, 1968–72); Giovanni Matteo Ferrari da Gradi, *Practica, seu Commentaria in Nonum Rasis ad Almansorem* (Venice: Iuntas, 1560), 370–89; Philippus Theophrastus Bombastus von Hohenheim [Paracelsus], "On the Diseases That Deprive Man of His Reason," in *Volumen Medicinae Paramirum*, trans. Kurt F. Leidecker (Baltimore: Johns Hopkins Press, 1949); Ambroise Paré (1517?–90), *Workes of That Famous . . . Chirurgion . . .*, trans. Thomas Johnson (London: R. Cotes and Young, 1634), 634–39; Robert Burton, *The Anatomy of Melancholy*, ed. F. Dell and Paul J. Smith (New York: Farrar and Rinehart, 1927), 353–57; Giulio Cesare Claudini, *Responsionum et Consultationem Medicinalium Tomus Unicus* (Frankfurt: Lazari Zetzneri, 1607), 402; William Harvey, *Anatomical Exercitations, concerning the Generation of Living Creatures . . .* (London: James Young for Octavian Pulleyn, 1653), 501–2; Nathaniel Highmore, *De Passione Hysterica et Affectione Hypochondriaca* (Oxford: A. Lichfield; R. Davis, 1660), Estevaõ Rodrigues de Castro, *Syntaxis Praedictionum Medicarum* (Lyons: Phil. Borde; Arnaud et Cl. Rigaud, 1661); Abraham Zacuto [Zacutus Lusitanus], *Praxis Medica Admiranda* (London: Ioannem; Huguetan Antonium, 1637),11, 13, 35, 40, 42, 46, 176–80, 252–66, 277–83, 289–95; Gregor Horst, *Dissertationem . . . Inauguralem de Mania . . . Publicae Censura* (Giessen: Frederic Karger's widow, 1677), 9–18; Bernard Mandeville, *A Treatise of the Hypochondriack and Hysteric Passions* (Hildesheim, 1711; reprint New York: G. Olms, 1981); Hermann Boerhaave, *Praelectiones Academicae de Morbis Nervorum Curant* (Leiden: Van Eems, 1761; reprint Leiden: Brill, 1959), 11, 144–45, 284–85, 290, 292, 370; William Cullen, *First Lines of the Practice of Physic* (Edinburgh: Bell, Bradfute, 1791), 98–115; Philippe Pinel, *A Treatise on Insanity*, trans. D. D. Davis (1806; facsimile reprint New York: Hafner, 1962), 7–45, 229–65; Franz Josef Gall, *Anatomie et physiologie du système nerveuse en général* (Paris: F. Schoell, 1810–19), 85–164; Auguste Élisabeth Philogène Tripier, *Leçons cliniques sur les maladies de femmes* (Paris: Octave Doin, 1883),

347–51; and Pierre Briquet, *Traité clinique et thérapeutique de l'hystérie* (Paris: J. B. Baillière, 1859), 111–38, 289–91, 409–12, 535–613.

3. The standard histories of the disease are Ilsa Veith, *Hysteria: The History of a Disease* (Chicago: University of Chicago Press, 1965); Alan Krohn, *Hysteria: The Elusive Neurosis* (New York: International Universities Press, 1978); Dewey Ziegler and Paul Norman, "On the Natural History of Hysteria in Women," *Diseases of the Nervous System* 15 (1967): 301–36; Henri Cesbron, *Histoire critique de l'hystérie* (Paris: Asselin et Houzeau, 1909); and Glafira Abrikosova, *L'hystérie aux XVIIe et XVIIIe siècles (étude historique)* (Paris: Steinheil, 1897). More recent works include Phillip R. Slavney, *Perspectives on "Hysteria"* (Baltimore: Johns Hopkins University Press, 1990), and George Wesley, *A History of Hysteria* (Washington, D.C.: University Press of America, 1979).

4. Donald E. Greydanus, "Masturbation; Historic Perspective," *New York State Journal of Medicine* 80, no. 12 (1980): 1892–96; E. H. Hare, "Masturbatory Insanity: The History of an Idea," *Journal of Mental Science* 108 (1962): 2–25; John Francis Wallace Meagher, *A Study of Masturbation and Its Reputed Sequelae* (New York: William Wood, 1924); E. H. Smith, "Signs of Masturbation in the Female," *Pacific Medical Journal*, February 1903, 78–83; Wilhelm Stekel, "Disguised Onanism (Masked Masturbation)," *American Journal of Urology and Sexology* 14, no. 7 (1918): 289–307.

5. For a survey of this research, see Donald Symons, *The Evolution of Human Sexuality* (New York: Oxford University Press, 1979), 75–92.

6. On the treatment of hysteria and chlorosis by midwives, see Nicolaas Fonteyn [Nicolaus Fontanus, fl. 1630], *The Womans Doctour* (London: John Blage and Samuel Howes, 1652), B4–7, 45; Jakob Rueff [1500–1558], *The Expert Midwife* (London: E. Griffin for S. Burton, 1637), bk. 6, chap. 8; Nicholas Culpeper [1616–54], *A Directory for Midwives* (London: Peter Cole, 1651), 94–95, 110–11; John Pechey [1655–1716], *A General Treatise of the Diseases of Maids, Big-Bellied Women, Child-Bed Women, and Widows* (London: Henry Bonwick, 1696), A3, B13–14; and his *Compleat Midwife's Practice Enlarged*, 5th ed. (1698), 230–33.

7. Franklin H. Martin, *Electricity in Diseases of Women and Obstetrics* (Chicago: W. T. Keener, 1892), 225–32; Franklin Benjamin Gottschalk, *Practical Electro-therapeutics* (Hammond, Ind.: F. S. Betz, 1908), 282; Gottschalk, *Static Electricity, X-ray and Electro-vibration: Their Therapeutic Application* (Chicago: Eisele, 1903), 137–39; Anthony Matijaca, *Principles of Electro-medicine, Electro-surgery and Radiology* (Tangerine, Fla.: Benedict Lust, 1917), 134–36; and Vibrator Instrument Company, *The Chattanooga Vibrator* (Chattanooga, Tenn.: VIC, 1904), 3.

8. Highmore, *De Passione Hysterica*, 76–77: "Necnon in lusu illo puerorum, quo una manu pectus perfricare, altera frontem percutere conantur."

9. Russell Thacher Trall, *The Health and Diseases of Women* (Battle Creek, Mich.: Health Reformer, 1873), 7–8, 31, and John Butler, *Dr. John Butler's Electro-massage Machine or Electric Manipulator for Curing Diseases at Home* (New York: Butler Electric Massage, 1889), 21.

10. Andrew Scull and Diane Favreau, "'A Chance to Cut Is a Chance to Cure': Sexual Surgery for Psychosis in Three Nineteenth Century Societies," *Research in Law, Deviance and Social Control* 8 (1986): 3–39; see also Hare, "Masturbatory Insanity," 10, and Vern Bullough, "Technology for the Prevention of 'Les Maladies Produites par la Masturbation,'" *Technology and Culture* 28, no. 4 (1987): 828–32.

11. For counterarguments to the view of "woman as physician's victim," see Regina Morantz, "The Lady and Her Physician," in *Clio's Consciousness Raised*, ed. M. Hartman and L. Banner (New York: Harper Torchbooks, 1974), 38–53.

12. Judith Brown has suggested that the absence of penetration in most lesbian activity accounts for its having been largely ignored in Western legal history. See Brown, *Immodest Acts: The Life of a Lesbian Nun in Renaissance Italy* (New York: Oxford University Press, 1986), 6–20.

13. See, for example, Celia Roberts et al., "Faking It: The Story of 'Ohh!'" *Women's Studies International Forum* 18, nos. 5–6 (1995): 531 n. 7.

14. Alfred Charles Kinsey, *Sexual Behavior in the Human Female* (Philadelphia: Saunders, 1953), and Shere Hite, *The Hite Report on Female Sexuality* (New York: Macmillan, 1976). Note also popular treatments of this subject such as Judith Schwartz, "Straight Talk about Orgasm," *Redbook* March (1994), 75. For earlier references to this subject see, for example, John Pechey, *The Compleat Midwife's Practice Enlarged*, 5th ed. (1698), 32; Culpeper, *Directory for Midwives*, 28; and an unusual mid-twentieth-century text, Alfred Henry Tyrer, *Sex Satisfaction and Happy Marriage* (New York: Emerson Books, 1948), 85, 115. A more conventional source is Marie Stopes, *Married Love: A New Contribution to the Solution of Sex Difficulties* (New York: Eugenics, 1931), 74.

15. Havelock Ellis, "The Sexual Impulse in Women," in *Studies in the Psychology of Sex*, vol. 1 (New York: Random House, 1940). A popular medical advice author of the 1970s, David Reuben follows more recent (but equally androcentric) conventions by using the expression "orgasmic impairment" to avoid what he considers to be the more judgmental "frigid." See Reuben, *Any Woman Can! Love*

and Sexual Fulfillment for the Single, Widowed, Divorced . . . and Married (New York: D. McKay, 1971), 25–56.

16. Joseph Frank Payne, *Thomas Sydenham* (New York: Longman, Green, 1900), 143.

17. Barbara Ehrenreich and Deirdre English, *Complaints and Disorders: The Sexual Politics of Sickness* (Old Westbury, N.Y.: Feminist Press, 1973), 15–44.

18. See, for example, Sophie Lazarsfeld, *Woman's Experience of the Male*, 9th ed. (London: Encyclopedic Press, 1967), 123–66.

19. For an especially notable example of this perspective, see Edmund Bergler and William S. Kroger, *Kinsey's Myth of Female Sexuality* (New York: Grune and Stratton, 1954), 7, 35, 70, 76, 94–95.

20. After at least two millennia of efforts to produce female orgasm before or during male orgasm in coitus, a study has suggested that conception is aided by female orgasm from one to forty-five minutes after ejaculation by the male. See Beth Livermore, "Why Women's Orgasms Matter," *Self* 16, no. 2 (1994): 56; F. Bryant Furlow and Randy Thornhill, "The Orgasm Wars," *Psychology Today*, January–February 1996, 42–46; and Michael Segell, "Great Performances," *Esquire* (January 1996), 30.

21. W. C. M. Schultz et al., "Vaginal Sensitivity to Electric Stimuli: Theoretical and Practical Implications," *Archives of Sexual Behavior* 18, no. 2 (1989): 87–95.

22. There are some who, like Juvenal in his *Satire on Women* (late first century A.D.), mention it for the purpose of condemning the supposed depravity of the female sex.

23. Such as Richardson's *Pamela* (1740), Tolstoy's *Anna Karenina* (1876), and Flaubert's *Madame Bovary* (1856).

24. For examples, see Symons, *Evolution of Human Sexuality*, 85–92; Helen Rodnite Lemay, "Human Sexuality in Twelfth- through Fifteenth-Century Scientific Writings," in *Sexual Practices and the Medieval Church*, ed. Vern L. Bullough and James Brundage (Buffalo, N.Y.: Prometheus Books, 1982), 204; Edward Bliss Foote, *Dr. Foote's Home Cyclopedia of Popular Medical, Social and Sexual Science* (New York: Murray Hill, 1901), 550, 1133, 1150; Robert Taylor, *A Practical Treatise on Sexual Disorders of the Male and Female*, 3d ed. (New York: Lea Brothers, 1905), 404, 410–13; and Smith Baker, "The Neuropsychical Element in Conjugal Aversion," *Journal of Nervous and Mental Disease* 19 (September 1892): 669–81.

25. Thomas Laqueur, *Making Sex: Body and Gender from the Greeks to Freud* (Cambridge: Harvard University Press, 1990), 34–35.

26. Michel Foucault, *The History of Sexuality*, vol. 1, *An Introduction* (New York: Random House, 1978), 104.

27. Jean-Michel Oughourlian, *The Puppet of Desire: The Psychology of Hysteria, Possession and Hypnosis*, trans. Eugene Webb (Stanford, Calif.: Stanford University Press, 1991), 145; on neurasthenia see John S. Haller, "Neurasthenia: The Medical Profession and the 'New Woman' of the Late Nineteenth Century," *New York State Journal of Medicine* 71 (February 15, 1971): 474.

28. Edward Haller Shorter, "Paralysis: The Rise and Fall of a 'Hysterical' Symptom," *Journal of Social History* 19, no. 4 (1986): 549–82.

29. Gall, *Anatomie et physiologie du système nerveux*, 85–164, and A. F. A. King, "Hysteria," *American Journal of Obstetrics* 24, no. 5 (1891): 513–32.

30. There is, however, at least one case of such an injury to a hysteric at the Salpêtrière. See Christopher G. Goetz, Michel Bonduelle, and Toby Gelfand, *Charcot: Constructing Neurology* (New York: Oxford University Press, 1995), 191.

31. Joan Jacobs Brumberg, *Fasting Girls: The Emergence of Anorexia Nervosa as a Modern Disease* (Cambridge: Harvard University Press, 1988), 67–70, 107, 115–20, 143.

32. Roberta Satow, "Where Has All the Hysteria Gone?" *Psychoanalytic Review* 66 (1979–80): 463–73. Martha Noel Evans argues that the disease survives, at least in France, in the form of disorders now called spasmophilia and anorexia, formerly diagnosed as hysteria. See Evans, *Fits and Starts: A Genealogy of Hysteria in Modern France* (Ithaca: Cornell University Press, 1991), 223–42.

33. Owsei Temkin, *Galenism; Rise and Decline of a Medical Philosophy* (Ithaca: Cornell University Press, 1973).

34. Paré, *Workes*, 634, 945.

35. As in Robert L. Dickinson and Henry H. Pierson, "The Average Sex Life of American Women," *Journal of the American Medical Association* 85 (1925): 1113–17; see also Harland William Long, *Sane Sex Life and Sane Sex Living: Some Things That All Sane People Ought to Know about Sex Nature and Sex Functioning* (New York: Eugenics, 1937), 125–27.

36. Among those who did, the most notable are Highmore, *De Passione Hysterica*, 76–78, and Tripier, *Leçons cliniques*, 350–51. Audrey Eccles discusses some

other forthright authors in *Obstetrics and Gynaecology in Tudor and Stuart England* (London: Croom Helm, 1982), 79–82, as do Danielle Jacquart and Claude Thomasset in *Sexuality and Medicine in the Middle Ages*, trans. Matthew Adamson (Princeton: Princeton University Press, 1988), 170.

37. Two of many examples are William Acton [1813–75], *The Functions and Disorders of the Reproductive Organs in Childhood, Youth, Adult Age and Advanced Life, Considered in Their Physiological, Social, and Moral Relations* (Philadelphia: Blakiston, 1865), 133, and Richard von Krafft-Ebing, *Psychopathia Sexualis: A Medico-forensic Study* (1886; reprint New York: G. P. Putman's Sons, 1965), 33, 55, 248. An overview of this literature appears in Carl N. Degler, "What Ought to Be and What Was," *American Historical Review* 79 (1974): 1467–90.

38. Peter Gay, *The Education of the Senses*, vol. 1 of *The Bourgeois Experience: Victoria to Freud* (New York: Oxford University Press, 1984), 103, 264, 478–82.

39. Laqueur, *Making Sex*, 233. "Frigidity" in men is also defined in the context of coitus. See Robert Knight, "Functional Disturbances in the Sexual Life of Men: Frigidity and Related Disorders," *Bulletin of the Menninger Clinic* 7, no. 1 (1943): 25–35.

40. Editorial in *Lancet*, 1869, quoted in Lynda Nead, *Myths of Sexuality: Representations of Women in Victorian Britain* (Oxford: Basil Blackwell, 1988): 21; C. Bigelow, *Sexual Pathology: A Practical and Popular Review of the Principal Diseases of the Reproductive Organs* (Chicago: Ottaway and Colbert, 1875), 36, 78, 109; and William Goodell, *Lessons in Gynecology*, 3d ed. (Philadelphia: Davis, 1890), 541, 565–70.

41. It has been observed that this is a fundamental difficulty with the Masters and Johnson research results. William H. Masters, *Human Sexual Response* (Boston: Little, Brown, 1966). Bergler and Kroger, in *Kinsey's Myth of Female Sexuality*, 48, claim that there is no scientific or statistical objection to declaring 80 to 90 percent of the female population abnormal.

42. For example, Mary Gove Nichols, *Experience in Water-Cure* (New York: Fowlers and Wells, 1850), 10–68; Nichols, *Lectures to Women on Anatomy and Physiology* (New York: Harper, 1846), 244–48; and Wilhelm Griesinger, *Mental Pathology and Therapeutics*, trans. C. Lockhart Robinson and James Rutherford (London: New Sydenham Society, 1867), 202.

43. Roger Blake, *Sex Gadgets* (Cleveland: Century, 1968), 33–46, and Akbar Del Piombo, *The Erotic Tool* (New York: Olympia Press, 1971), 38–39.

44. See, for example, the views of female orgasm in Howard S. Levy and Akira Ishihara, *The Tao of Sex: The "Essence of Medical Prescriptions (Ishimpo),"* 3d ed. rev. (Lower Lake, Calif.: Integral, 1989), a translation of a tenth-century work by Tamba Yasuyori, a Chinese physician who lived in Japan; and Al-Sayed Haroun ibn Hussein Al-Makhzoumi [fl. A.D. 1152?], *The Fountains of Pleasure*, trans. Hatem El-Khalidi (New York: Dorset Press, 1970), 65–76.

45. American Psychiatric Association, *Mental Disorders Diagnostic Manual* (Washington, D.C.: APA, 1952).

46. Carol Tavris and Carole Wade, *The Longest War: Sex Differences in Perspective*, 2d ed. (San Diego: Harcourt Brace Jovanovich, 1984), 92–96.

47. Joseph Mortimer Granville, *Nerve-Vibration and Excitation as Agents in the Treatment of Functional Disorders and Organic Disease* (London: J. and A. Churchill, 1883). See also the Weiss model of Mortimer Granville's design at the Bakken Library and Museum of Electricity in Life, Minneapolis, accession number 82.100. Trade catalog sources include Wappler Electric Manufacturing Company, *Wappler Cautery and Light Apparatus and Accessories*, 2d ed. (New York: Wappler Electric, 1914); Sam J. Gorman, *Electro-therapeutic Apparatus*, 10th ed. (Chicago: Sam J. Gorman, 1912); and Manhattan Electrical Supply Company, *Catalogue Twenty-six: Something Electrical for Everybody* (New York: MESCO, n.d.).

48. Some works that clarify these distinctions are Paul Tabori, *The Humor and Technology of Sex* (New York: Julian Press, 1969), 444; Helen Singer Kaplan, "The Vibrator: A Misunderstood Machine," *Redbook*, May 1984, 34; Mimi Swartz, "For the Woman Who Has Almost Everything," *Esquire*, July 1980, 56–63; "The Great Playboy Sex-Aids Road Test," *Playboy* 25, no. 3 (1978): 135–37, 208–9; and Joani Blank, *Good Vibrations* (Burlingame, Calif.: Down There Press, 1989), 6–25.

49. Zacuto, *Praxis Medica Admiranda*, 265–66.

50. Samuel Monell, *A System of Instruction in X-Ray Methods and Medical Uses of Light, Hot Air, Vibration and High Frequency Currents* (New York: E. R. Penton, 1903), 591–99.

51. Hieronymus Eusebius [Saint Jerome], *Select Letters of Saint Jerome*, trans. F. A. Wright (Cambridge: Harvard University Press, 1933), letters 45.5, 107.8, 11, 117.6.

52. See, for examples, Emmet Murphy, *Great Bordellos of the World* (London: Quartet Books, 1983), 55, 69. On masturbation with water, see Eugene Halpert, "On a Particular Form of Masturbation in Women: Masturbation with Water,"

Journal of the American Psychoanalytic Association 21 (1973): 526, and J. Aphrodite [pseud.], *To Turn You On: Thirty-nine Sex Fantasies for Women* (Secaucus, N.J.: Lyle Stuart, 1975), 83–91.

53. Barry Cunliffe, "The Roman Baths at Bath: The Excavations, 1969–1975," *Britannia* 7 (1976): 1–32.

54. Tobias Smollett, *An Essay on the External Use of Water,* ed. Claude E. Jones (London, 1752; reprint Baltimore: Johns Hopkins Press, 1935), 55–78.

55. Such as those in Tompkins and Chemung Counties, New York, in the mid-nineteenth century. Samuel A. Cloyes, *The Healer: The Story of Dr. Samantha S. Nivison and Dryden Springs, 1820–1915* (Ithaca, N.Y.: DeWitt Historical Society of Tompkins County, 1969), and "Medical Milestones," *Chemung Historical Journal* (Elmira, N.Y.) 32, no. 2 (1986): 3617–23. The *Water Cure Journal* cites many examples of women owners, co-owners, and resident physicians.

56. Henri Scoutetten, *De l'eau, ou De l'hydrothérapie* (Paris: P. Bertrand, 1843), 239–41.

57. Herbert Ant and Walter S. McClellan, "Physical Equipment for Administration of Health Resort Treatment," *Journal of the American Medical Association* 123 (November 13, 1943): 69–99.

58. For examples, see Good Health Publishing Company, *Twentieth Century Therapeutic Appliances* (Battle Creek, Mich.: Good Health, 1909), and Simon Baruch, *The Principles and Practice of Hydrotherapy: A Guide to the Application of Water in Disease* (New York: William Wood, 1897).

59. For examples of fees, see Charles B. Thorne, "The Watering Spas of Middle Tennessee," *Tennessee History Quarterly* 29, no. 4 (1970–71): 321–59, and J. A. Irwin, *Hydrotherapy at Saratoga* (New York: Casell, 1892). Other hydrotherapeutic spas are described in Edward C. Atwater and Lawrence A. Kohn, "Rochester and the Water Cure," *Rochester History* 32 (1970): 1–24; John Bell [1796–1872], *On Baths and Mineral Waters* (Philadelphia: H. H. Porter, 1831); Augustus P. Biegler, *The Rochester Lake View Water-Cure Institution* (Rochester, N.Y., 1851); Carl Bridenbaugh, "Baths and Watering Places of Colonial America," *William and Mary Quarterly* 3 (1946): 151–81; Edward Bulwer-Lytton, *Confessions of a Water-Patient*, 3d ed. (London: H. Baillière, 1847); Susan Evelyn Cayleff, "Wash and Be Healed: The Nineteenth-Century Water-Cure Movement, 1840–1900. Simple Medicine and Women's Retreat" (Ph.D. diss., Brown University, 1983); Jane B. Donegan, *Hydropathic Highway to Health: Women and*

Water-Cure in Antebellum America (Westport, Conn.: Greenwood Press, 1986); and Edward W. Fitch, *Mineral Waters of the United States and American Spas* (Philadelphia: Lea and Feibiger, 1927).

60. Alfred Levertin, *Dr. G. Zander's Medico-mechanical Gymnastics: Its Method, Importance and Applications* (Stockholm: P. A. Norstedt, 1893).

61. "All physicians agree that every family should have an Electric Battery in their house," advertisement by United States Battery Agency (Brooklyn, N.Y.), *Dorcas Magazine* 7 (September 15, 1889). Edward Trevert Bubier, *Electro-therapeutic Handbook* (New York: Manhattan Electrical Supply Company, 1900), 86; and N. A. Cambridge, "Electrical Apparatus Used in Medicine before 1900," *Proceedings of the Royal Society of Medicine* 70, no. 9 (1977): 635–41.

62. Taylor wrote voluminously and invented tirelessly. His major works include *Paralysis and Other Affections of the Nerves: Their Cure by Transmitted Energy and Special Movements* (New York: American Book Exchange, 1880); *Massage* (New York: Fowler and Wells, 1884); *Diseases of Women* (Philadelphia: G. McClean, 1871); *Health for Women* (New York: John B. Alden, 1883); *Health for Women: Showing the Causes of Feebleness and the Local Diseases Resulting Therefrom, with Full Directions for Self-Treatment*, 12th ed. (New York: Health Culture, 1923); "March 21, 1875. Improvement in medical rubbing apparatus," U.S. Patent 175,202, application filed May 17, 1875; *Mechanical Aids in the Treatment of Chronic Forms of Disease* (New York: Rodgers, 1893); *Pelvic and Hernial Therapeutics* (New York: J. B. Alden, 1885); and "Movement Cure," U.S. Patent 263,625, application filed June 19, 1882. Figure 3 is from *Pelvic and Hernial Therapeutics*.

63. Mortimer Granville, *Nerve-Vibration and Excitation*, 57.

64. Noble Murray Eberhart, *A Brief Guide to Vibratory Technique*, 4th ed. rev. and enl. (Chicago: New Medicine Publication, 1915), 59.

65. Vibrator Instrument Company, *Chattanooga Vibrator*.

66. Monell, *System of Instruction in X-Ray Methods*, 595.

67. Mary Lydia Hastings Arnold Snow, *Mechanical Vibration and Its Therapeutic Application* (New York: Scientific Authors, 1904).

68. Richard J. Cowen, *Electricity in Gynecology* (London: Baillière, Tindall and Cox, 1900), 73–74; George J. Engelmann, "The Use of Electricity in Gynecological Practice," *Gynecological Transactions* 2 (1886): 134; Hermon E. Hoyd, "Electricity in Gynecological Practice," *Buffalo Medical and Surgical Journal*, May

1890; George Betton Massey, *Conservative Gynecology and Electrotherapeutics* (Philadelphia: F. A. Davis, 1898); and Mary Cushman Rice, *Electricity in Gynecology* (Chicago: Laing, 1909).

69. Alfred Dale Covey, *Profitable Office Specialities* (Detroit: Physicians Supply Company, 1912), 79–95; Samuel Spencer Wallian, *Rhythmotherapy: A Discussion of the Physiologic Basis and Therapeutic Potency of Mechano-vital Vibration, to Which Is Added a Dictionary of Diseases with Suggestions as to the Technic of Vibratory Therapeutics* (Chicago: Ouellette Press, 1906); and Wallian, "The Undulatory Theory in Therapeutics," *Medical Brief* (Chicago), May–June 1905.

70. *American Magazine*, 1916; see also 75, no. 2 (1912); 75, no. 3 (1913); and 75, no. 7 (1913): 127. Other such advertisements appeared in *Needlecraft*, September 1912, 23; *Home Needlework Magazine*, October 1908, 479, and October 1915, 45; *Hearst's*, January 1916, 67, February 1916, 154, April 1916, 329, June 1916, 473; and *National Home Journal*, September 1909, 15. An advertisement soliciting male door-to-door sales representatives for vibrators appeared in *Modern Priscilla*, April 1913, 60.

71. "Such Delightful Companions! Star Electrical Necessities," 1922, reproduced in Edgar R. Jones, *Those Were the Good Old Days* (New York: Fireside Books, 1959). See also "A Gift That Will *Keep* Her Young and Pretty: Star Home Electric Massage," *Hearst's International*, December 1921, 82.

72. Examples of advertisements for these devices include "Agents! Drop Dead Ones! Awake! Grab this new invention! The 20th century wonder, Blackstone Water Power Vacuum Massage Machine," *Hearst's*, April 1916, 327; "10 pennies lead ten people to get $32,000.00!" advertisement for Allen's portable bath apparatus, *Men and Women*, May 1910, 80; "Corbin vacuo-masseur. For facial massage. A flesh builder. Price $1.50." *Woman's Home Companion* 36 (May 1909): 57; "Ediswan Domestic Appliances. Use more electrical appliances in your home," advertisement for pneumatic massage pulsator, *Electrical Age for Women* (Glasgow) 2 (January 7, 1932), inside front cover; booklet, *Vibration: Nature's Great Underlying Force for Health, Strength and Beauty* (Detroit: Golden Manufacturing Company, [ca. 1905]); Good Health, *Twentieth Century Therapeutic Appliances;* Hamilton-Beach Manufacturing Company (Racine, Wisc.), "What would you give for a perfect, healthy body?" 1913 advertisement for New Life vibrator, reproduced in Jones, *Those Were the Good Old Days;* Lambert Snyder Company (New York), "This marvelous health vibrator for man, woman and child; relieves all suffering; cures disease," *Modern Woman* 11 (April 5, 1907): 170; Lindstrom-Smith Company, advertisement, *Technical World*, 1928; *Popular Mechanics*, December 1928; Professor Rohrer's Institute of Beauty Culture, *Rohrer's Illus-*

trated Book of Scientific Modern Beauty Culture (New York: Professor Rohrer's Institute, n.d.); and Leslie Smith, *Vibratory Technique and Directions for Treatment with White Cross Electric Vibrator* (Chicago: National Stamping and Electrical Works, 1917).

73. Sears, Roebuck and Company, *Electrical Goods: Everything Electrical for Home, Office, Factory and Shop* (Chicago: Sears, Roebuck, 1918), 4.

74. "Development in Electrical Apparatus during 1917," *Electrical Review*, January 5, 1918; A. Edkins, "Prevalent Trend of Domestic Appliance Market," *Electrical World*, March 30, 1918, 670–71; "Electrical Appliance Sales during 1926: Tabulation," *National Electric Light Association Bulletin* 14 (February 1927): 119; "Electrical devices for the household," advertisement, *Scientific American* 96 (January 1907): 95; "Electrical Exhibits and Demonstrations in Wanamakers' New York Store," *Electrical World*, November 3, 1906; "Electromedical Apparatus for Domestic Use," *Electrical Review of London* 99 (October 22, 1926): 682; and C. Frederick, "Selling Small Electrical Appliances," *Electrician* 99 (November 11, 1927): 590–91.

75. Robert T. Francoeur, *Becoming a Sexual Person* (New York: John Wiley, 1982), 37.

Chapter 2 Female Sexuality as Hysterical Pathology

1. On this point see Eliot Slater, "What Is Hysteria?" in *Hysteria*, ed. Alec Roy (New York: John Wiley, 1982), 39–40.

2. Susan B. Anthony is said to have regarded male behavior at sports events as evidence that men were too emotional to be allowed to vote.

3. Edward Haller Shorter, "Paralysis: The Rise and Fall of a 'Hysterical' Symptom," *Journal of Social History* 19, no. 4 (1986): 549–82.

4. George Wesley, *A History of Hysteria* (Washington, D.C.: University Press of America, 1979), 6.

5. For example, Phillip R. Slavney, *Perspectives on "Hysteria"* (Baltimore: Johns Hopkins University Press, 1990), and Carroll Smith-Rosenberg, "The Hysterical Woman: Sex Roles and Role Conflict in Nineteenth Century America," *Social Research* 39 (winter 1972): 652–78.

6. Apparent loss of consciousness for a brief interval after orgasm has been noted in some women. See Linda Wolfe, *The Cosmo Report* (New York: Arbor House, 1981), 125.

7. Jean-Michel Oughourlian, *The Puppet of Desire: The Psychology of Hysteria, Possession and Hypnosis*, trans. Eugene Webb (Stanford, Calif.: Stanford University Press, 1991), 145.

8. Ann Ellis Hanson, "Hippocrates: Diseases of Women," *Signs* 1 (1975): 567–84.

9. Aulus Cornelius Celsus, *On Medicine*, trans. W. G. Spencer (Cambridge: Harvard University Press, 1935), vol. 1, chap. 4, 20.307.

10. Soranus of Ephesus, *Gynecology*, trans. Owsei Temkin (Baltimore: Johns Hopkins Press, 1956), 140–70.

11. Aretaeus Cappadox, *The Extant Works of Aretaeus the Cappadocian*, ed. and trans. Francis Adams (London: Sydenham Society, 1856), 300–301, and Aretaeus, "On the Causes and Symptoms of Acute Diseases," in ibid., bk. 2, chap. 2.

12. Galen of Pergamon, *De Locis Affectis*, trans. Rudolph Siegel (New York: S. Karger, 1976), bk. 6, 2.39.

13. Äetius of Amida, "Tetrabiblion," trans. James Ricci, in *The Gynaecology and Obstetrics of the Sixth Century A.D.* (Philadelphia: Blakiston, 1950).

14. Mustio [Moschion], *La "Gynaecia" di Muscione*, ed. and trans. Rino Radicchio (Pisa: Giardini, 1970), 122.

15. The masculine paranoia implicit in this view of the uterus really does not deserve comment.

16. *Medieval Woman's Guide to Health*, trans. Beryl Rowland (Kent, Ohio: Kent State University Press, 1981), 87.

17. Danielle Jacquart and Claude Thomasset, *Sexuality and Medicine in the Middle Ages*, trans. Matthew Adamson (Princeton: Princeton University Press, 1988), 170. The authors cite several other medieval medical authorities who advocate vulvular massage as therapy, among them Albertus Magnus and John of Gaddesden.

18. Avicenna (Ibn Sina, 980–1037), *Liber Canonis* (1507; reprint Hildesheim: G. Olms, 1964), 3.20.1:44.

19. Nancy G. Siraisi, *Medieval and Early Renaissance Medicine: An Introduction to Knowledge and Practice* (Chicago: University of Chicago Press, 1990), 115–23, 128, 135.

20. Helen Rodnite Lemay, *Women's Secrets: A Translation of Pseudo-Albertus Magnus's "De Secretis Mulierum" with Commentaries* (Saratoga Springs: State University of New York Press, 1992), 6, 130–35.

21. Giovanni Matteo Ferrari da Gradi, *Practica, seu Commentaria in Nonum Rasis ad Almansorem* (Venice: Iuntas, 1560), 389: "Haec itaque passio, cum primum, evenerit, curanda est. Cuius curatio est, ut pedes fortiter, fricenter & ligenter & cucurbitula magna sumini superponanter. & Obstetrici quoque precipiatur, ut digitum oleo, bene redolente, in circuitu oris vulvae, dum est intus, bene commoveat."

22. Philippus Theophrastus Bombastus von Hohenheim [Paracelsus], "On the Diseases That Deprive Man of His Reason," in *Volumen Medicinae Paramirum*, trans. Kurt F. Leidecker (Baltimore: Johns Hopkins Press, 1949).

23. Ambroise Paré, *Workes of That Famous . . . Chirurgion . . .*, trans. Thomas Johnson (London: R. Cotes and Young, 1634), 634.

24. Paré, *Workes*, 945.

25. Audrey Eccles, *Obstetrics and Gynaecology in Tudor and Stuart England* (London: Croom Helm, 1982), 82.

26. Eccles, *Obstetrics and Gynaecology*, 79.

27. Robert Burton, *The Anatomy of Melancholy*, ed. Floyd Dell and Paul Jordan Smith (New York: Farrar and Rinehart, 1927), 355.

28. Giulio Cesare Claudini, *Responsionum et Consultationem Medicinalium Tomus Unicus* (Frankfurt: Lazari Zetzneri, 1607), 402.

29. G. Rattray Taylor, *Sex in History*, quoted in Richard Cavendish, ed., *Man, Myth and Magic* (New York: Marshall Cavendish, 1970), 193.

30. Michael MacDonald, *Mystical Bedlam: Madness, Anxiety and Healing in Seventeenth-Century England* (New York: Cambridge University Press, 1981), 39. MacDonald does not mention the great antiquity of this concept.

31. Abraham Zacuto, *Praxis Medica Admiranda* (London: Ioannem-Antonium Huguetan, 1637), 265–66.

32. Nicolaas Fonteyn, *The Womans Doctour* (London: John Blage and Samuel Howes, 1652), B4–6.

33. John Pechey, *The Compleat Midwife's Practice Enlarged*, 5th ed. (1698), 232–33.

34. Thomas Sydenham, "Epistolary Dissertation [on Hysteria]," in *The Works of Thomas Sydenham*, trans. R. G. Latham, vol. 2 (London: Sydenham Society, 1848), and Joseph Frank Payne, *Thomas Sydenham* (New York: Longman, Green, 1900), 143.

35. William Harvey, *Anatomical Exercitations concerning the Generation of Living Creatures* (London: James Young for Octavian Pulleyn, 1653), 501–2.

36. William Harvey, "On Parturition," in *The Works of William Harvey*, trans. Robert Willis (London: Sydenham Society, 1847; reprint New York: Johnson, 1965), 542–45.

37. Nathaniel Highmore, *De Passione Hysterica et Affectione Hypochondriaca* (Oxford: A. Lichfield-R. Davis, 1660), 76–78.

38. See, for example, Thomas Willis (1621–75), *Affectionum Quae Dicuntur Hystericae et Hypochondriacae Vindica contra Reponsionem Epistolarum Nathaniel Highmore* (London, 1681); published in English as his *Essay on the Pathology of the Brain and Nervous Stock* (London: J. Dring, 1681), 77–81. Willis's objections were primarily to Highmore's hypothesis that hysteria was a disease of the blood, not to the form of treatment. Culpeper, an older contemporary, apparently disapproved of traditional treatments for hysteria. See Nicholas Culpeper (1616–54), *A Directory for Midwives* (London: Peter Cole, 1651), 94–95, 110–11.

39. Hermann Boerhaave, *Praelectiones Academicae de Morbis Nervorum Curant* (Leiden: Van Eems, 1761; reprint Leiden: Brill, 1959), 290–92.

40. Bernard Mandeville, *A Treatise of the Hypochondriack and Hysteric Passions* (Hildesheim, 1711; reprint New York: G. Olms, 1981). For a modern reference to female equestrian orgasm, see Jane McIlvaine McClary, *A Portion for Foxes* (New York: Simon and Schuster, 1972), 162–63.

41. Robert H. MacDonald, "The Frightful Consequences of Onanism: Notes on the History of a Delusion," *Journal of the History of Ideas* 28, no. 3 (1967): 425.

42. The work cited is Albrecht von Haller's *Disputationes ad Morborum Historiam et Curationem Facientes* (Lausanne: Marci-Michael Bousquet, 1757–60).

43. William Cullen, *First Lines of the Practice of Physic* (Edinburgh: Bell, Bradfute, 1791), 4:96–115.

44. Accounts of this appear in David Hume, *Enquiries concerning Human Understanding and concerning the Principles of Morals*, 3d ed. rev. (1777; reprint Oxford: Clarendon Press, 1975), 124–25, and Louis Basile Carré de Montgeron, *La verité des miracles operés par l'intercession de M. de Paris* (Utrecht: Libraires de Compagnie, 1737). Charles K. Mills remarks darkly that "great immorality prevailed in the secret meetings of the believers"; see "Hysteria," in *A System of Practical Medicine*, vol. 5, *Diseases of the Nervous System*, ed. William Pepper and Louis Starr (Philadelphia: Lea Brothers, 1886), 224.

45. Charles MacKay, *Extraordinary Popular Delusions and the Madness of Crowds* (London, 1841; reprint New York: Farrar, Straus and Giroux, 1972), 318, 323; see also Geoffrey Sutton, "Electric Medicine and Mesmerism," *Isis* 72, no. 263 (1981): 375–92.

46. Franz Josef Gall, *Anatomie et physiologie du système nerveux en général* (Paris: F. Schoell, 1810–19), 3:86: "La crise ne manquoit jamais de se terminer par une évacuation qui avoit lieu avec tressaillements de la volupté, et dans une véritable extase; après quoi, elle restoit sans attaques pendant quelques temps."

47. See, for example, Roger Thompson, *Sex in Middlesex: Popular Mores in a Massachusetts County, 1649–1699* (Amherst: University of Massachusetts Press, 1986), 42.

48. Jan Goldstein, *Console and Classify: The French Psychiatric Profession in the Nineteenth Century* (New York: Cambridge University Press, 1987), 324.

49. Thomas Stretch Dowse, *Lectures on Massage and Electricity in the Treatment of Disease* (Bristol: John Wright, 1903), 181.

50. The anemia hypothesis is set forth in Karl Figlio, "Chlorosis and Chronic Disease in Nineteenth-Century Britain: The Social Constitution of Somatic Illness in a Capitalist Society," *Social History* 3 (1978): 167–97. See also Robert Hudson, "The Biography of a Disease: Lessons from Chlorosis," *Bulletin of the History of Medicine* 51 (1977): 448–63.

51. Thomas Laycock (1812–76), *A Treatise on the Nervous Diseases of Women* (London: Longman, Orme, Brown, 1840), 140–42; quoted in Figlio, "Chlorosis," 178.

52. Mary Gove Nichols, *Lectures to Women on Anatomy and Physiology* (New York: Harper, 1846), 181.

53. George M. Beard, *Sexual Neurasthenia [Nervous Exhaustion]* (New York: E. B. Treat, 1884).

54. John S. Haller Jr., "Neurasthenia: The Medical Profession and the 'New Woman' of the Late Nineteenth Century," *New York State Journal of Medicine* 71 (February 15, 1971): 474.

55. Quoted in Haller, "Neurasthenia," 478.

56. F. G. Gosling, *Before Freud: Neurasthenia and the American Medical Community, 1870–1910* (Urbana: University of Illinois Press, 1987), 52, 114.

57. Gosling, *Before Freud*, 52. For a discussion of male neurasthenia, see E. Anthony Rotundo, *American Manhood: Transformations in Masculinity from the Revolution to the Modern Era* (New York: Basic Books, 1993), 187–89.

58. Ernest Jones, *Papers on Psychoanalysis*, 2d ed. (London: Baillière, Tindall and Cox, 1918), 559; quoted in E. H. Hare, "Masturbatory Insanity: The History of an Idea," *Journal of Mental Science* 108, no. 452 (1962): 9.

59. R. J. Culverwell, *Porneiopathology: A Popular Treatise on Venereal Diseases of the Male and Female Genital System* (New York: J. S. Redfield, 1844), 165.

60. Robert Brudenell Carter, *On the Pathology and Treatment of Hysteria* (London: John Churchill, 1853); Charles Delucena Meigs, *Woman: Her Diseases and Remedies*, 3d ed. (Philadelphia: Blanchard and Lea, 1854), 65.

61. Meigs, *Woman*, 474.

62. James Manby Gully, *The Water-Cure in Chronic Diseases: An Exposition* (New York: Fowler and Wells, 1854), 185–87. For Gully's public relations difficulties, see William E. Swinton, "The Hydrotherapy and Infamy of Dr. James Gully," *Canadian Medical Association Journal*, no. 123 (December 12, 1980): 1262–64.

63. Curran Pope, *Practical Hydrotherapy: A Manual for Students and Practitioners* (Cincinnati: Lancet-Clinic, 1909), 181, 510–12.

64. Pierre Briquet, *Traité clinique et thérapeutique de l'hystérie* (Paris: J. B. Baillière, 1859), vii, 1–10, 37, 111, 116–17, 137–38, 291, 535, 543, 570, 613.

65. Briquet, *Traité*, 123–26, 612–22.

66. Wilhelm Griesinger, *Mental Pathology and Therapeutics* (London: New Sydenham Society, 1867; reprint New York: Hafner, 1965), 179–81.

67. Russell Thacher Trall, *The Health and Diseases of Women* (Battle Creek, Mich.: Health Reformer, 1873), 7–8.

68. Ann Douglas Wood, "The Fashionable Diseases: Women's Complaints and Their Treatment in Nineteenth-Century America," in *Clio's Consciousness Raised*, ed. Mary Hartman and Lois W. Banner (New York: Harper Torchbooks, 1974), 3.

69. Albert H. Hayes, *The Physiology of Woman and Her Diseases, or Woman, Treated of Physiologically, Pathologically and Esthetically* (Boston: Peabody Medical Institute, 1869), 250–51.

70. C. Bigelow, *Sexual Pathology: A Practical and Popular Review of the Principal Diseases of the Reproductive Organs* (Chicago: Ottaway and Colbert, 1875), 78–85.

71. Auguste Élisabeth Philogène Tripier, *Leçons cliniques sur les maladies de femmes: Thérapeutique générale et applications de l'électricité à ces maladies* (Paris: Octave Doin, 1883), 350–51.

72. Tripier, *Leçons cliniques*, 46–47.

73. Richard von Krafft-Ebing, *Psychopathia Sexualis: A Medico-forensic Study* (1886; reprint New York: G. P. Putnam's Sons, 1965), 33, 64, 77.

74. Jules Philippe Falret, *Études cliniques sur les maladies mentales et nerveuses* (Paris: Librairie Baillière, 1890), 500–502.

75. Gilles de la Tourette, *Traité clinique et thérapeutique de l'hystérie paroxistique* (Paris: Plon, 1895), 1:433, 461: "L'acte sexuel a été pour l'hystérique plus qu'une désillusion: elle ne le comprend pas; il lui inspire des répugnances insurmontables."

76. Désiré Magloire Bourneville, *Iconographie photographique de la Salpêtrière* (Paris: Progrès Médicale, 1878), 1:8, 2:97–193: "Th. pousse un cri plus ou moins prolongé: Oue! Oue! et jette brusquement la tête sur la ligne médiane (Pl. III C). Après un court repos, surviennent les mouvements de balancement: Th. fléchit violemment le tronc, puis le rejette in arrière, ces mouvement se répètent cinq ou six fois avec grand rapidité. Puis, le corps se met en arc en conserve cette position durant quelques seconds. On observe ensuite quelques mouvements legères du bassin . . . Ensuite, la scène change. A . . . se soulève, se recouche, pousse de cris de joie, rit, s'agite, a quelques mouvements lubriques, et tombe dans un vulve et de la hanche droite."

77. William Goodell, *Lessons in Gynecology*, 3d ed. (Philadelphia: Davis, 1890), 539–66.

78. Franklin H. Martin, *Electricity in Diseases of Women and Obstetrics* (Chicago: W. T. Keener, 1892), 221–23.

79. Friedrich Eduard Bilz, *The New Natural Method of Healing* (London: A. Bilz, 1898), 683–84.

80. William H. Dieffenbach, *Hydrotherapy* (New York: Rebman, 1909), 238.

81. A. F. A. King, "Hysteria," *American Journal of Obstetrics* 24, no. 5 (1891): 517–22.

82. Sigmund Freud, "Charcot," in *Complete Psychological Works*, vol. 3, 1893–1899, ed. James Strachey and Anna Freud (London: Hogarth Press, 1962), 16–21.

83. Freud, *Complete Psychological Works*, vol. 14, quoted in Neil Hertz, "Dora's Secrets, Freud's Techniques," in *In Dora's Case: Freud—Hysteria—Feminism*, ed. Charles Bernheimer and Claire Kahane (New York: Columbia University Press, 1985), 238–39.

84. Michel Foucault, *The History of Sexuality*, vol. 1, *An Introduction* (New York: Random House, 1978), 112.

85. Jean-Martin Charcot, *Clinical Lectures on Certain Diseases of the Nervous System*, trans. E. P. Hurd (Detroit: G. S. Davis, 1888).

86. Georges Guillain, *J.-M. Charcot, 1825–1893: His Life and Work*, trans. Pearce Bailey (New York: Hoeber, 1959), 134.

87. Quoted in Ilsa Veith, *Hysteria: The History of a Disease* (Chicago: University of Chicago Press, 1965), 267.

88. Editor's note to Freud's *Complete Psychological Works*, 2:xi.

89. Sigmund Freud, "The Aetiology of Hysteria" (1896), in *Complete Psychological Works*, 3:189–208.

90. Fritz Wittels, *Freud and His Time* (New York: Grosset and Dunlap, 1931), chap. 7, "The Hysterical or Primary Type," 222.

91. Havelock Ellis, "Auto-erotism," in *Studies in the Psychology of Sex* (1910; New York: Random House: 1940), 1:225.

92. Christopher Goetz, Michel Bonduelle, and Toby Gelfand, *Charcot: Constructing Neurology* (New York: Oxford University Press, 1995), 172–216. There was much disagreement about paralysis as a symptom among Freud's and Charcot's contemporaries. See, for example, Charles K. Mills, "Hysteria," 236–37.

93. Wilhelm Reich, *Genitality in the Theory and Therapy of Neurosis*, trans. Philip Schmitz (1927; reprint New York: Farrar, Straus and Giroux, 1980), 54–93.

94. Wesley, *History of Hysteria*, 2.

95. George Swetlow, "Hysterics as Litigants," *Bulletin of the Medical Society of the County of Kings* (New York), June 1953; reprinted in Cambria (Pennsylvania) County Medical Society, *Medical Comment*, September 1953, 3–9.

96. Carroll Smith-Rosenberg, "Hysterical Woman," and Smith-Rosenberg and Charles Rosenberg, "The Female Animal: Medical and Biological Views of Woman and Her Role in Nineteenth-Century America," *Journal of American History* 60 (1973): 332–56.

97. Barbara Ehrenreich and Deirdre English, *Complaints and Disorders: The Sexual Politics of Sickness* (Old Westbury, N.Y.: Feminist Press, 1973), 31. Hysteria is discussed on 15–44, esp. 39.

98. Foucault, *History of Sexuality*, 1:104.

99. Peter Gay, *The Education of the Senses*, vol. 1 of *The Bourgeois Experience: Victoria to Freud* (New York: Oxford University Press, 1984), 264. There are discussions of hysteria on 103 and 478–82.

100. Oughourlian, *Puppet of Desire*, 149.

101. Gay, *Education of the Senses*, 197.

Chapter 3 "My God, What Does She Want?"

1. Donald Symons, *The Evolution of Human Sexuality* (New York: Oxford University Press, 1979), 85.

2. William H. Masters, *Human Sexual Response* (Boston: Little, Brown, 1966).

3. Symons, *Evolution of Human Sexuality*, 87. He cites Alfred Charles Kinsey, *Sexual Behavior in the Human Female* (Philadelphia: Saunders, 1953); see 163 and 189.

4. Carol Tavris and Carole Wade, *The Longest War: Sex Differences in Perspective*, 2d ed. (San Diego: Harcourt Brace Jovanovich, 1984), 92–93.

5. This question is not original to me. See Shere Hite, *The Hite Report on Male Sexuality* (New York: Ballantine Books, 1981), 680.

6. Paul Robinson, *The Modernization of Sex: Havelock Ellis, Alfred Kinsey, William Masters, and Virginia Johnson* (New York: Harper and Row, 1976), 137.

7. The social and legal implications of this view have been explored in detail by Susan Brownmiller, *Against Our Will: Men, Women and Rape* (New York: Simon and Schuster, 1975).

8. The Ptolemaic system is illustrated and described in Otto Neugebauer, *The Exact Sciences in Antiquity*, 2d ed. (1957; reprint New York: Dover, 1969), 191–206; Giorgio de Santillana, *The Origins of Scientific Thought* (New York: Mentor Books, 1961), 251–53; and many other works on Greek science and mathematics.

9. Examples are numerous. For American medical authors, see Nancy Sahli, *Women and Sexuality in America: A Bibliography* (Boston: G. K. Hall, 1984).

10. Thomas Laqueur, *Making Sex: Body and Gender from the Greeks to Freud* (Cambridge: Harvard University Press, 1990), 34–35.

11. Mirko D. Grmek, "The Harm in Broad Beans: Legend and Reality," in *Diseases in the Ancient Greek World* (Baltimore: Johns Hopkins University Press, 1988), 210.

12. Laqueur, *Making Sex*, 49–51.

13. Franz Josef Gall, *Anatomie et physiologie du système nerveux en général* (Paris: F. Schoell, 1810–19), 3:91. For an example of a modern medical text on this subject, see Edwin B. Steel and James H. Price, *Human Sex and Sexuality*, 2d ed. (New York: Dover, 1988), 244. A fictional, but documented, comment appears in Gay Courter's novel *The Midwife's Advice* (New York: Signet, 1994), 100, 301, 376–77, and author's note, 713–16, on European folk and modern medical research on the observed correlation, in some populations, between female orgasm and the conception of male children.

14. Danielle Jacquart and Claude Thomasset, *Sexuality and Medicine in the Middle Ages* (Princeton: Princeton University Press, 1988), 67.

15. Helen Rodnite Lemay, "Human Sexuality in Twelfth- through Fifteenth-Century Scientific Writings," in *Sexual Practices and the Medieval Church*, ed. Vern L. Bullough and James Brundage (Buffalo, N.Y.: Prometheus Books, 1982), 204.

16. Audrey Eccles, *Obstetrics and Gynaecology in Tudor and Stuart England* (London: Croom Helm, 1982), 28–30, 68.

17. Ambroise Paré, *Workes of That Famous . . . Chirugion . . .* , trans. Thomas Johnson (London: R. Cotes and Young, 1634), 945–46.

18. Abraham Zacuto, *Praxis Medica Admiranda* (London: Ioannem-Antonium Huguetan 1637), 260: "Horribilis affectio est, & odiosa: nam concubitum, & conceptionem impedit."

19. Franz Josef Gall, *Sur les fonctions du cerveau* (Paris: J. B. Baillière, 1825), 3:235.

20. Nathaniel Highmore, *De Passione Hysterica et Affectione Hypochondriaca* (Oxford: A. Lichfield-R. Davis, 1660), 5–6, 41–45, 71.

21. William Cullen, *First Lines of the Practice of Physic* (Edinburgh: Bell, Bradfute, 1791), 3:46–47, 4:105.

22. Laqueur, *Making Sex*, 218.

23. Carroll Smith-Rosenberg and Charles Rosenberg, "The Female Animal: Medical and Biological Views of Woman and Her Role in Nineteenth-Century America," *Journal of American History* 60 (1973): 348–49.

24. C. Bigelow, *Sexual Pathology: A Practical and Popular Review of the Principal Diseases of the Reproductive Organs* (Chicago: Ottaway and Colbert, 1875), 36, 78, 109.

25. William Goodell, *Lessons in Gynecology*, 3d ed. (Philadelphia: Davis, 1890), 541, 565–70.

26. Edward Bliss Foote, *Dr. Foote's Home Cyclopedia of Popular Medical, Social and Sexual Science* (New York: Murray Hill, 1901), 550, 1133, 1150. Foote considered this exchange to be of vital importance to health and believed that men and women improved each other's health simply by standing close together fully dressed. He also asserted, "as a man's rights man!" the right of men to be treated by physicians of the opposite sex, and thus endorsed the active recruitment of women doctors.

27. Richard von Krafft-Ebing, *Psychopathia Sexualis: A Medico-forensic Study* (1896; New York: G. P. Putnam's Sons, 1965), 33, 55, 248.

28. John S. Haller and Robin Haller, *The Physician and Sexuality in Victorian America* (Urbana: University of Illinois Press, 1973), 99.

29. G. Kolischer, "Sexual Frigidity in Women," *American Journal of Obstetrics* 52, no. 3 (1905): 414–16.

30. Gilles de la Tourette, *Traité clinique et thérapeutique de l'hystérie paroxistique* (Paris: Plon, 1895), 1:461.

31. Theodore Gaillaird Thomas, *A Practical Treatise on the Diseases of Women*, 6th ed. (Philadelphia: Lea Brothers, 1891), 124–25.

32. Smith Baker, "The Neuropsychical Element in Conjugal Aversion," *Journal of Nervous and Mental Disease* 19, no. 9 (1892): 669–81.

33. Havelock Ellis, *Studies in the Psychology of Sex*, vol. 1 (New York: Random House, 1940), 245–70.

34. N. Cooke, *Satan in Society* (Cincinnati: C. F. Vent, 1871), 91–105, 112.

35. Bigelow, *Sexual Pathology*, 33; Charles H. Hendricks, "The Sewing Machine Problem as Seen through the Pages of the *American Journal of Obstetrics and Diseases of Women and Children*, 1868–1873," *Obstetrics and Gynecology* 26 (1965):

453–54, and "Influence of Sewing Machine on Female Health," *New Orleans Medical and Surgical Journal* 20 (November 1867): 359–60.

36. Krafft-Ebing, *Psychopathia Sexualis*, 498; A. Coffignon, *Paris vivant: La corruption à Paris* (Paris: Librarie Illustrée, [1888?]).

37. Thomas Low Nichols, *The Curse Removed: A Statement of Facts Respecting the Efficacy of Water-Cure in the Treatment of Uterine Disease and the Removal of the Pains and Perils of Pregnancy and Childbirth* (New York: Water-Cure Journal, 1850), 12.

38. E. H. Smith, "Signs of Masturbation in the Female," *Pacific Medical Journal*, February 1903, 76–83. See also Robert Taylor, A *Practical Treatise on Sexual Disorders of the Male and Female*, 3d ed. (New York: Lea Brothers, 1905), 418.

39. R. Pearsall, *The Worm in the Bud: The World of Victorian Sexuality* (New York: Macmillan, 1969), 204.

40. Mary Gove Nichols, *Experience in Water-Cure* (New York: Fowlers and Wells, 1850), 61–68. See also Jayme A. Sokolow, *Eros and Modernization: Sylvester Graham, Health Reform, and the Origins of Victorian Sexuality in America* (Rutherford, N.J.: Fairleigh Dickinson University Press, 1983), 127.

41. Russell Thacher Trall, *The Hydropathic Encyclopedia* (New York: Fowlers and Wells, 1852), 443–47, and Trall, *Nervous Debility; The Nature, Causes, Consequences, and Hygienic Treatment of Invalids, Suffering from Prematurely Exhausted Vitality* (New York: Davies and Kent, 1861), 15–16.

42. Russell Thacher Trall, *The Health and Diseases of Women* (Battle Creek, Mich.: Health Reformer, 1873), 31.

43. George M. Beard, *Sexual Neurasthenia [Nervous Exhaustion]* (New York: E. B. Treat, 1884), 120, 201–5.

44. Ilsa Veith, *Hysteria: The History of a Disease* (Chicago: University of Chicago Press, 1965), 100–101.

45. Ornella Moscucci, *The Science of Woman: Gynaecology and Gender in England, 1800–1929* (New York: Cambridge University Press, 1990), 112–27.

46. Robert Brudenell Carter, *On the Pathology and Treatment of Hysteria* (London: John Churchill, 1853), 69.

47. Virginia G. Drachman, "The Loomis Trial: Social Mores and Obstetrics in the Mid-Nineteenth Century," in *Women and Health in America: Historical Readings*, ed. Judith Walzer Leavitt (Madison: University of Wisconsin Press,

1984), 167–68. See also Wilhelm Griesinger, *Mental Pathology and Therapeutics*, trans. C. Lockhart Robinson and James Rutherford (London: New Sydenham Society, 1867), 202. For a contemporary medical description of the technique, see Thomas, *Practical Treatise on the Diseases of Women*, 78–79.

48. James Marion Sims, *The Story of My Life* (New York: D. Appleton, 1884), 231.

49. Dianne Grosskopf, *Sex and the Married Woman* (New York: Simon and Schuster, 1983), 121, found vaginal insertion as a primary masturbatory technique in 11 percent of her sample; Kinsey, *Sexual Behavior in the Human Female*, 189, found 20 percent.

50. Donald E. Greydanus, "Masturbation: Historic Perspective," *New York State Journal of Medicine* 80, no. 12 (1980): 1893.

51. Jeffrey Moussaieff Masson, *The Assault on Truth: Freud's Suppression of the Seduction Theory* (New York: Farrar, Straus and Giroux, 1987), 84–91, and Madelon Sprengnether, "Enforcing Oedipus," in *In Dora's Case: Freud—Hysteria—Feminism*, ed. Charles Bernheimer and Claire Kahane (New York: Columbia University Press, 1985), 265.

52. Taylor, *Practical Treatise*, 404, 410–13.

53. Jan Goldstein, *Console and Classify: The French Psychiatric Profession in the Nineteenth Century* (New York: Cambridge University Press, 1987), 374.

54. Decimus Junius Juvenal, *The Satires of Juvenal*, trans. Rolfe Humphries (Bloomington: Indiana University Press, 1958), 67–68, 81.

55. D'Emilio and Freedman comment on this in the context of Puritanism. John D'Emilio and Estelle Freedman, *Intimate Matters: A History of Sexuality in America* (New York: Harper and Row, 1988), 28.

56. Adam Raciborski, *De la puberté chez la femme* (Paris: J. B. Baillière, 1844), 486.

57. Carl W. Degler, *At Odds: Women and the Family in America from the Revolution to the Present* (New York: Oxford University Press, 1980), 255.

58. William Alexander Hammond, *Sexual Impotence in the Male and Female* (Detroit: G. S. Davis, 1887), 300.

59. Hermann Fehling, *Lehrbuch der Frauenkrankheiten* (Stuttgart: Enke, 1893). The translation is by Havelock Ellis, who quotes him on p. 195 of "The Sexual Impulse in Women," in *Studies in the Psychology of Sex*.

60. Ellis, "Sexual Impulse in Women," 191.

61. They are also consistent with Ann Landers's findings of 72 percent with a sample size of about 100,000 readers in 1985, and with those of Linda Wolfe, with a figure of 71 percent among 106,000 women. See Wolfe, *The Cosmo Report* (New York: Arbor House, 1981), 129.

62. Sophie Lazarsfeld, *Woman's Experience of the Male* (London: Encyclopedic Press, 1967), 308.

63. D'Emilio and Freedman, *Intimate Matters*, 71.

64. Clelia Duel Mosher, *The Mosher Survey: Sexual Attitudes of Forty-five Victorian Women* (New York: Arno Press, 1980); D'Emilio and Freedman, *Intimate Matters*, 80–81. See also Regina Markell Morantz, "Making Women Modern: Middle Class Women and Health Reform in Nineteenth Century America," *Journal of Social History* 10 (1977): 490–507, and Edward Shorter, *A History of Women's Bodies* (New York: Basic Books, 1982), 9–16.

65. Laqueur, *Making Sex*, 206. Lynda Nead says, "The ideal of female virtue was an important element in the feminist attack on the double standard . . . . The feminist campaign . . . colluded in the propagation of a single legitimate sexuality." See Nead, *Myths of Sexuality: Representations of Women in Victorian Britain* (Oxford: Basil Blackwell, 1988), 23.

66. Laqueur, *Making Sex*, 233.

67. Auguste Élisabeth Philogène Tripier, *Leçons cliniques sur les maladies de femmes: Thérapeutique générale et applications de l'électricité à ces maladies* (Paris: Octave Doin, 1883), 347: "Des observations si non décisives du moins assez multipliées, m'ont laissé la conviction que l'orgasme vénérien est lié, chez la femme, au concours de deux ordres, au moins de sensations les unes clitoridiennes, les autres utér-ovariennes; que la synergie de ces deux ordres d'impression est nécessaire à la production de l'orgasme physiologique; enfin, que ces deux modes de sensibilité peuvent être lésés ensemble ou séparément."

68. Edmund Bergler and William S. Kroger, *Kinsey's Myth of Female Sexuality* (New York: Grune and Stratton, 1954), 7.

69. Bergler and Kroger, *Kinsey's Myth*, 48.

70. Paul H. Gebhard et al., *The Sexuality of Women* (New York: Stein and Day, 1970), 121.

71. Robert L. Dickinson and Henry H. Pierson, "The Average Sex Life of American Women," *Journal of the American Medical Association* 85 (1925): 1113–17.

72. Jeanne Warner, "Physical and Affective Dimensions of Female Sexual Response and the Relationship to Self-Reported Orgasm," in *International Research in Sexology: Selected Papers from the Fifth World Congress*, ed. Harold Lief and Zwi Hoch (New York: Praeger, 1984), 91–94; Joseph Bohlen et al., "The Female Orgasm: Pelvic Contractions," *Archives of Sexual Behavior* 11, no. 5 (1982): 367–86.

73. Grosskopf, *Sex and the Married Woman*, 35–43.

74. Gebhard et al., *Sexuality of Women*, 122.

75. Ann Landers, "What 100,000 Women Told Ann Landers," *Reader's Digest* 127 (August 1985): 44; Charles Leerhsen, "Ann Landers and 'the Act,'" *Newsweek* 105 (January 28, 1985): 76–77; and Ann Landers, "Sex: Why Women Feel Short-Changed," *Family Circle*, June 11, 1985, 85, 132–36. Landers's readers were asked, "Would you be content to be held close and treated tenderly and forget about 'the act'?"

76. Peter Gay, *The Education of the Senses*, vol. 1 of *The Bourgeois Experience: Victoria to Freud* (New York: Oxford University Press, 1984), 133–44.

77. Carl N. Degler, "What Ought to Be and What Was: Women's Sexuality in the Nineteenth Century," *American Historical Review* 79 (1974): 1467–90; see esp. 1470–71, 1474–75, 1479, 1481–84, 1487.

78. Marie Carmichael Stopes, *Married Love: A New Contribution to the Solution of Sex Difficulties* (New York: Eugenics, 1931), 32.

Chapter 4 "Inviting the Juices Downward"

1. Samuel Howard Monell, *A System of Instruction in X-Ray Methods and Medical Uses of Light, Hot-Air, Vibration and High Frequency Currents* (New York: E. R. Denton, 1903), 591.

2. Samuel Spencer Wallian, *Rhythmotherapy: A Discussion of the Physiologic Basis and Therapeutic Potency of Mechano-vital Vibration, to Which Is Added a Dictionary of Diseases with Suggestions as to the Technic of Vibratory Therapeutics* (Chicago: Ouellette Press, 1906), 56.

3. For a discussion of these saws, see D. L. Simms, "Water-Driven Saws in Late Antiquity," *Technology and Culture* 26 (April 1985): 275–76.

4. Carl Sandzen, *An Article on Vibratory Massage* (Philadelphia: Keystone Electric, 1904), 63. Sandzen says only that the device was intended "as a means of counteracting a sedentary mode of living."

5. See, for example, Wiliam Sermon (1629?-79), *The Ladies Companion, or The English Midwife* (London: Edward Thomas, 1671), 8.

6. Ambroise Paré, *Workes of That Famous . . . Chirurgion . . .*, trans. Thomas Johnson (London: R. Cotes and Young, 1634).

7. Audrey Eccles, *Obstetrics and Gynaecology in Tudor and Stuart England* (London: Croom Helm, 1982), 11–16.

8. Theodore Gaillaird Thomas, *A Practical Treatise on the Diseases of Women*, 6th ed. (Philadelphia: Lea Brothers, 1891), 394.

9. A. Sigismond Weber, *Traitement par l'électricité et le massage* (Paris: Alex Coccoz, 1889), 73–80.

10. George Betton Massey, *Conservative Gynecology and Electro-therapeutics* (Philadelphia: F. A. Davis, 1898), 70–71.

11. Silas Weir Mitchell, *Fat and Blood: An Essay on the Treatment of Certain Forms of Neurasthenia and Hysteria* (Philadelphia: J. B. Lippincott, 1877), 54–55.

12. Thomas Low Nichols, *The Curse Removed: A Statement of Facts Respecting the Efficacy of Water-Cure in the Treatment of Uterine Disease and the Removal of the Pains and Perils of Pregnancy and Childbirth* (New York: Water-Cure Journal, 1850), 15.

13. Jacqueline S. Wilke, "Submerged Sensuality: Technology and Perceptions of Bathing," *Journal of Social History* 19 (summer 1986): 649–64. For a highly decorous discussion of Greek baths, see J. H. Croon, "Hot Springs and Healing Gods," *Mnemosyne* 20 (1967): 225–46.

14. Anthony J. Papalas, "Medicinal Bathing in Mineral Springs in Fifth Century BC Greece," *Clio Medica* 16, nos. 2–3 (1981): 81–82. On animal trails, see Charles B. Thorne, "The Watering Spas of Middle Tennessee," *Tennessee History Quarterly* 29, no. 4 (1970–71): 321–59.

15. Apparently this was even true in upright Quaker areas of Pennsylvania, although the Quaker elders disapproved of their members' visiting spas. See Carol Shiels Roark, "Historic Yellow Springs: The Restoration of an American Spa," *Pennsylvania Folklife* 24, no. 1 (1974): 30–35. Roark reports that six hundred people a day visited Yellow Springs in the summertime during the 1770s. The modern spas at, for example, Saratoga Springs, New York, and Yverdon-les-Bains, Switzerland, still have facilities nearby for sports and gambling.

16. Francis Power Cobbe, "The Medical Profession and Its Morality," *Modern Review* 2 (1881): 306, 316.

17. Georges Simenon, *The Bells of Bicêtre* (New York: Harcourt, Brace and World, 1963), 39. For accounts of life at English spas in the seventeenth century, see Celia Fiennes, *Illustrated Journeys c1682–c1712*, ed. Christopher Morris (London: Webb and Bower, 1982), 18, 45, 92, 125, 158. Fiennes points out that many mineral springs were regarded by Catholics as holy places despite their reputation for social license.

18. Iris Murdoch, *The Philosopher's Pupil* (New York: Viking, 1983), 16–31.

19. Hilary Evans, *Harlots, Whores and Hookers: A History of Prostitution* (New York: Dorset Press, 1979), 47, and Alan Anderson, *Vanishing Spas* (Dorchester, England: Friary Press, 1974), 11, 70–71, 90.

20. J. A. Cosh, "Rheumatism Treatment Centres in Britain—Bath, Ancient and Modern," *Annals of Physical Medicine* 10 (November 1969): 167–71.

21. A. Cianconi, "La cure termali ginecologiche nei 'Fontes Clusini' in periodo medievale," in *Atti, Twenty-first International Congress of the History of Medicine*, Siena, Italy, 1968 (Rome, 1969), 1:56–67.

22. Tobias Smollett, *An Essay on the External Use of Water*, ed. Claude E. Tolles (London, 1752; Baltimore: Johns Hopkins Press, 1935), 55, 60, 65, 71, 78.

23. On women's straightforward enjoyment of hydrotherapeutic establishments, independent of any sexual pleasure of the kind I am arguing for, see Susan Evelyn Cayleff, "Wash and Be Healed: The Nineteenth-Century Water-Cure Movement, 1840–1900. Simple Medicine and Women's Retreat" (Ph.D. diss., Brown University, 1983).

24. Robin Price, "Hydropathy in England, 1840–70," *Medical History* 25, no. 3 (1984): 271–72.

25. Sebastien Kneipp, *Pfarrer Kneipp's volf stümliche . . . Vorträge über feine . . .* (Wörishofen: Hartmann, 1894), fig. 16.

26. J. A. Irwin, *Hydrotherapy at Saratoga* (New York: Cassell, 1892), 112, 123–25, 246–48. Readers uncertain about the meaning of "textural unctuosity" may avail themselves of the mineral bathing facilities still operating at Saratoga, Greenbriar, and other locations in the United States and Europe.

27. R. J. Lane, *Life at the Water Cure: Facts and Fancies* (London: Horsell, 1851), 56, 58, 61, 102, 230.

28. G. H. Doudney, *The Water Cure in the Bedroom* (Bristol: John Wright, 1891), 13.

29. Joseph Buckley, *Recollections of the Late John Smedley and the Water Cure* (1888; Matlock, England: Arkwright Society, 1973), introductory essay by D. A. Barton and p. 36.

30. Barry Cunliffe, "The Roman Baths at Bath: The Excavations, 1969–1975," *Britannia* 7 (1976): 1.

31. W. B. Oliver, "The Blood and Circulation," *Lancet*, June 27, 1896; quoted in Simon Baruch, *The Principles and Practice of Hydrotherapy: A Guide to the Application of Water in Disease* (New York: William Wood, 1897), 215. The *Lancet* had been highly skeptical of hydrotherapy before 1852; see Price, "Hydropathy in England," 274.

32. Gilles de la Tourette, *Maladies du système nerveux* (Paris: Plon, 1898), 174.

33. Walter S. McClellan, "Hydrotherapy and Balneotherapy," in *Modern Medical Therapy in General Practice* (New York: Williams and Wilkins, 1940), 431.

34. John Harvey Kellogg's *Rational Hydrotherapy* (Philadelphia: Davis, 1901) includes good illustrations of hydriatic equipment.

35. Patricia Spain Ward, *Simon Baruch: Rebel in the Ranks of Medicine, 1840–1921* (Tuscaloosa: University of Alabama Press, 1994), 231.

36. Alexander MacKay, "High Season in the 1840's," in *Western World, or Travels in the United States in 1846–47*, 2d ed., vol. 2 (Philadelphia: Lea and Blanchard, 1849); quoted in Roger Haydon, ed., *Upstate Travels: British Views of Nineteenth-Century New York* (Syracuse, N.Y.: Syracuse University Press, 1982), 110.

37. Marietta Holley, *Samantha at Saratoga, or Flirtin' with Fashion* (Philadelphia: Hubbard Brothers, 1887). This is also true of Edna Ferber's characters in *Saratoga Trunk* (New York: Fawcett Crest, 1969), 132–33.

38. Quoted in William L. Stone, *Reminiscences of Saratoga and Ballston* (New York: Virtue and Yorston, 1875), 161.

39. Harold Meeks, "Smelly, Stagnant and Successful: Vermont's Mineral Springs," *Vermont History* 47, no. 1 (1979): 5–20; Neil Pond, "Tennessee's Tyree Springs: The Most Celebrated Watering Place in the State," *Kentucky Folklore Record* 24, nos. 3–4 (1978): 64–73; and Ray Woodlief, "North Carolina's Mineral Springs," *North Carolina Medical Journal* 25 (1964): 159–64. On cold-water spas, see Estrellita Karsh, "Taking the Waters at Stafford Springs: The Role of the Willard Family in America's First Health Spa," *Harvard Library Bulletin* 28, no. 3 (1980): 264–81.

40. Edward C. Atwater and Lawrence A. Kohn, "Rochester and the Water Cure," *Rochester History* 32, no. 4 (1970): 6.

41. Predictably, these physicians left a wealth of bibliographic evidence of their activities. See Walter S. McClellan, "Collections on the History of Balneology in Saratoga Springs, NY," *Bulletin of the History of Medicine* 20, no. 4 (1946): 571–98.

42. Atwater, "Rochester and the Water Cure," 9–21.

43. Barbara Ehrenreich and Deirdre English, *Complaints and Disorders: The Sexual Politics of Sickness* (Old Westbury, N.Y.: Feminist Press, 1973), 42. See also illustrations of this technique in Buckley, *Recollections of the late John Smedley and the Water Cure*, unpaged illustrations, and Baruch, *Principles and Practice of Hydrotherapy*, 101.

44. Kathryn Kish Sklar, "All Hail to Pure Cold Water," in *Women and Health in America: Historical Readings*, ed. Judith Walzer Leavitt (Madison: University of Wisconsin Press, 1984), 252.

45. Abigail May, *Journal at Ballstown Springs, 1800*, transcribed from the original at the New York State Historical Association by Field Horne (Ballston Spa, N.Y.: Saratoga County Historical Society, 1982), 16–17.

46. May, *Journal*, 38.

47. Baruch, *Principles and Practice of Hydrotherapy*, 211–12, 366, 376–78.

48. Edward Johnson, *The Domestic Practice of Hydropathy* (New York: John Wiley, 1849), 76–77, 261–68.

49. Mary Louise Shew, *Water-Cure for Ladies* (New York: Wiley and Putnam, 1844), 135–36.

50. Mary Gove Nichols, *Experience in Water-Cure* (New York: Fowler and Wells, 1850), 15, 44, 61–62, and her *Lectures to Women on Anatomy and Physiology* (New York: Harper, 1846), 181, 244–48.

51. Thomas Low Nichols, *An Introduction to the Water-Cure* (New York: Fowler and Wells, 1850), 40–45.

52. James Manby Gully, *The Water-Cure in Chronic Diseases: An Exposition* (New York: Fowler and Wells, 1854), 185–87, 353.

53. William H. Dieffenbach, *Hydrotherapy* (New York: Rebman, 1909), 58, 238, 245.

54. Curran Pope, *Practical Hydrotherapy: A Manual for Students and Practitioners* (Cincinnati: Lancet-Clinic, 1909), 510–12.

55. Pope, *Practical Hydrotherapy*, 181, 185, 192.

56. Guy Hinsdale, *Hydrotherapy* (Philadelphia: W. B. Saunders, 1910), 224.

57. Shere Hite, *The Hite Report on Female Sexuality* (New York: Macmillan, 1976), 21, 53–55.

58. Linda Wolfe, *The Cosmo Report* (New York: Arbor House, 1981), 171.

59. For example, "Get this $1200 next month," Allen Portable Bath Apparatus advertisement, *Bohemian*, insert to 1909 volume, unpaged, and similar advertisement "10 Pennies Lead Ten People to get $32,000.00!" also for the Allen Portable Bath, *Men and Women*, May 1910, 80. A later incarnation of this technology appears in "New Amazing Portable Wall Shower," *Workbasket* 17, no. 11 (1952): 70.

60. Donald E. Greydanus, "Masturbation; Historic Perspective," *New York State Journal of Medicine* 80, no. 12 (1980): 1893–94; W. R. Miller and H. I. Lief, "Masturbatory Attitudes, Knowledge, and Experience: Data from the Sex Knowledge and Attitude Test (SKAT)," *Archives of Sexual Behavior* 5 (1976): 447.

61. J. Aphrodite [pseud.], *To Turn You On: Thirty-nine Sex Fantasies for Women* (Secaucus, N.J.: Lyle Stuart, 1975), 90.

62. Eugene Halpert, "On a Particular Form of Masturbation in Women: Masturbation with Water," *Journal of the American Psychoanalytic Association* 21 (1973): 526.

63. Two accounts of this method of masturbation are Jane Wallace, *Masturbation: A Woman's Handbook* (Bloomfield, N.J.: R. J. Williams, 1975), 23, and Boston Women's Health Book Collective, *The New Our Bodies, Ourselves: A Book by and for Women* (New York: Simon and Schuster, 1984), 168.

64. N. A. Cambridge, "Electrical Apparatus Used in Medicine before 1900," *Proceedings of the Royal Society of Medicine* 70, no. 9 (1977): 635–41. For an examples of electrets, see "The Only Electric Massage Roller," Dr. John Wilson Gibbs Company (New York), advertisement in *Cosmopolitan* 34, no. 1 (1902).

65. I owe this explanation of electrets to Al Kuhfeld, curator of the Bakken Library and Museum of Electricity in Life, which has a collection of these devices. For an example of an electric hairbrush, see "Free Christmas Offer . . . Dr. Scott's Electric Hair Brushes," Pall Mall Electric Company (New York), advertisement in *Needlecraft*, November 1924, 41.

66. Kevin Kane and Arthur Taub, "A History of Local Electrical Analgesia," *Pain* 1, no. 2 (1975): 127–34.

67. Audrey B. Davis, *Medicine and Its Technology: An Introduction to the History of Medical Instrumentation* (Westport, Conn.: Greenwood Press, 1981), 22.

68. For examples, see Auguste Vigouroux, *Étude sur la résistance électrique chez les mélancoliques* (Paris: J. Rueff, 1890); "Electricity the Renewer of Youth," *American Review of Reviews* 37 (June 1908): 732–33; T. Shueler, "Electricity and Light in Modern Medicine," *Scientific American*, suppl., 69 (April 2, 1910): 212–13; William John McRoberts, *Vibratory Rates Anatomical, Physiological, Pathological, Psychological and Dietetic as Worked out through "Streborcam" for "Streborcam" Technique in Detecting the Human Emanations in Diagnosing and Treating Diseases Utilizing Only the Ether . . .* (Hot Springs, S.D.: W. J. McRoberts, 1928); and George Lakhovsky, *La science et la bonheur, longevité, et immortalité par les vibrations* (Paris: Gauthier-Villars, 1930).

69. Albert Laquerrière, "Éxercise électriquement provoqué," paper presented at IIIe Congrès Internationale de Physiotherapie, 27 March–2 April 1910, 21–24.

70. Matthew J. Grier, "The Treatment of Some Forms of Sexual Debility by Electricity," paper presented at first annual meeting of the American Electro-therapeutic Association, Philadelphia, September 1891; reprinted from the *Times and Register*, November 21, 1891.

71. T. Robert Horton, *To Both Sexes of All Ages . . . Dr. Horton Cures Diseases of a Private Nature in an Incredibly Short Space of Time* (Sydney: McCarron, Stewart, n.d.), and "An Improved Electric Belt," *Scientific American* 68 (May 6, 1893): 277. For examples of the types of batteries sold to consumers, see T. Eaton and Company, "Electrical Sundries," *Catalogues for Spring and Summer; Fall and Winter* (1901; reprint Toronto: Musson, 1970), 118; Montgomery Ward and Company, "Electrical Goods," *Catalogue and Buyer's Guide No. 57* (spring and summer 1895; reprint New York: Dover, 1969), 214; and Sears, Roebuck and Company, "Department of Electric Belts," *Catalogue No. 111* (1902; reprint New York: Bounty Books, Crown, 1969), 475–76.

72. Richard von Krafft-Ebing, *Psychopathia Sexualis: a Medico-forensic Study* (1886; New York: G. P. Putnam's Sons, 1965), 114.

73. David V. Reynolds, "A Brief History of Electrotherapeutics," in *Neuroelectric Research: Electroneuroprosthesis, Electroanesthesia, and Nonconvulsive Electrotherapy*, ed. David V. Reynolds and Anita E. Sjoberg (Springfield, Ill.: Thomas, 1971), 6.

74. William Snowdon Hedley, *The Hydro-electric Methods in Medicine* (London: H. K. Lewis, 1892), 41–49.

75. International Correspondence Schools, *A System of Electrotherapeutics* (Scranton, Pa.: International Textbook, 1903), 4:40, 120–21; 5–7:113–19.

76. "Motor-Operated Therapeutic Machine," *Electrical World* 71 (March 2, 1918): 490.

77. George J. Engelmann, "The Use of Electricity in Gynecological Practice," *Gynecological Transactions* 11 (1886): 134.

78. Richard J. Cowen, *Electricity in Gynecology* (London: Baillière, Tindall and Cox, 1900), 74.

79. Herman E. Hoyd, "Electricity in Gynecological Practice," *Buffalo Medical and Surgical Journal*, May 1890, 5.

80. A. Lapthorn Smith, "Disorders of Menstruation," in *An International System of Electro-therapeutics*, ed. Horatio Bigelow (Philadelphia: F. A. Davis, 1894), G-159.

81. Franklin H. Martin, *Electricity in Diseases of Women and Obstetrics* (Chicago: W. T. Keener, 1892), 221.

82. Martin, *Electricity in Diseases of Women*, 232.

83. Havelock Ellis, "Auto-erotism," in *Studies in the Psychology of Sex*, vol. 1 (1910; New York: Random House, 1940), 168.

84. John Harvey Kellogg, "Electrotherapeutics in Chronic Maladies," paper presented at the International Electrical Congress, St. Louis, Mo., September 22, 1904; reprinted in *Modern Medicine*, October–November 1904, 8, 16.

85. John Butler, *Dr. John Butler's Electro-massage Machine for Curing Disease at Home. Glad Tidings for All, Men and Women. The Greatest Medical Discovery Ever Known* (New York: Butler Electro-massage, 1888), 19, 22, 34.

86. William Goodell also reported this desire to sleep after massage and electricity had been used to "promote the secretions." See Goodell, *Lessons in Gynecology* (Philadelphia: Davis, 1890), 539–40.

87. John Butler, *Electro-massage* (Philadelphia: Globe, 1880), 7–8, 14.

88. Health-Beauty Publishing Company, *Health-Beauty, or Common Sense Instead of Drugs* (New York: Health-Beauty, [ca. 1900]).

89. World's Columbian Exposition, *World's Columbian Exposition, Chicago, U.S.A, 1893; Classification and Rules, Department of Electricity* (Chicago: World's Columbian Exposition, 1893), 23.

90. John H. Girdner, "Healing by Electricity," *Munsey's Magazine* 29 (April 1903): 85.

91. John V. Shoemaker, "Electricity in the Treatment of Disease," *Scientific American*, suppl., 63 (January 5, 1907): 25924.

92. William H. Armstrong and Company, [*Catalogue of Medical Instruments*] (Indianapolis: Armstrong, 1901), 610–11.

93. For example, see Edward Trevert Bubier, *Electro-therapeutic Handbook* (New York: Manhattan Electrical Supply, [1900]), and Keystone Electric Company, *Illustrated Catalogue and Price List of Electrotherapeutic Appliances* (Philadelphia: Keystone Electric, [ca. 1903]). Wappler was another example; see Davis, *Medicine and Its Technology*, 22.

94. U.S. Bureau of the Census, *Census of Manufactures*, 1905, part 4, *Special Reports on Selected Industries* (Washington, D.C.: Government Printing Office, 1908), 216–17.

95. U.S. Bureau of the Census, *Census of Manufactures*, 1914, vol. 2, *Special Reports for Selected Industries and Detail Statistics for Industries, by States* (Washington, D.C.: Government Printing Office, 1919), 203.

96. U.S. Bureau of the Census, *Census of Manufactures*, 1947, vol. 2, *Statistics by Industry* (Washington, D.C.: Government Printing Office, 1949), 748. See John Liston, "Developments in the Electrical Industry during 1933: Electromedical Apparatus," *General Electric Review* 37 (January 1934): 40–41.

97. "All Physicians Agree that every family should have an Electric Battery in their house," United States Battery Agency (Brooklyn, N.Y.), advertisement in *Dorcas Magazine* 7, no. 1 (1889): v; and the same advertisement on the front flyleaf of *Conemaugh: A Graphic Story of the Johnstown Flood, from the Pens of the Journalists Who Were in the Valley* (New York: American News Company, 1889). See also electrotherapeutic devices in "Credit 18 months, installments, health, beauty, fine figure & complexions, drugs fail, new electricity succeeds. Home batteries. Free trial," Woman's Institute (Los Angeles), advertisement in *Ladies' World*, February 1898, 23, and "The only electric massage roller," Dr. John Wilson Gibb's Obesity Cure (New York), advertisement in *Cosmopolitan* 34, no. 1 (1902), unpaged advertising section.

98. "Oxydonor in the Home," Dr. H. Sanchez and Company (Detroit, Chicago, New York, and Montreal), advertisement in *Cosmopolitan* 34, no. 1 (1902), unpaged advertising section.

99. Western Merchandise and Supply Company, "Beauty for you Electric Massage," Home Electronic Massage Battery, advertisement, 1913, reproduced in *Those Were the Good Old Days*, ed. Edgar R. Jones (New York: Simon and Schuster, 1959), 186.

100. Master Electric Company, *The Master Violet Ray* (Chicago: Master Electric, n.d.), 2. The Bakken Library and Museum of Electricity in Life has some excellent examples of violet ray devices and their electrodes.

101. "Stop that Pain! with Violet Ray. Vibration Ozone Medical Electricity," Elco Electric Health Generators, Lindstrom and Company (Chicago), advertisement in *Popular Mechanics*, December 1928, advertising section, 4b.

102. Edward Ely Van de Warker, "Effects of Railroad Travel upon the Health of Women," *Georgia Medical Companion* 2 (1892): 192–206.

103. Soranus of Ephesus, *Gynecology*, trans. Owsei Temkin (Baltimore: Johns Hopkins Press, 1956), 140–41; Paré, *Workes*, 639, 948; Thomas Sydenham, *The Works of Thomas Sydenham*, trans. R. G. Latham (London: Sydenham Society, 1848), 2:116, 235; see also Ilsa Veith, *Hysteria: The History of a Disease* (Chicago: University of Chicago Press, 1965), 118.

104. Charles Delucena Meigs, *Woman: Her Diseases and Remedies*, 3d ed. (Philadelphia: Blanchard and Lea, 1854), 437.

105. Krafft-Ebing, *Psychopathia Sexualis*, 260–61, 466; George M. Beard, *Sexual Neurasthenia* (New York: E. B. Treat, 1884), 100; and John S. Haller and Robin M. Haller, *The Physician and Sexuality in Victorian America* (Urbana: University of Illinois Press, 1974), 185.

106. Somewhat paradoxically, there were also conditions allegedly caused by railroad travel called "railroad brain" and "railroad spine," which gave rise to numerous lawsuits in the nineteenth century. See Charles K. Mills, "Hysteria," in *A System of Practical Medicine*, vol. 5, *Diseases of the Nervous System*, ed. William Pepper and Louis Starr (Philadelphia: Lea Brothers, 1886), 225.

107. Charles William Malchow, *The Sexual Life: A Scientific Treatise Designed for Advanced Students and the Professions, Embracing the Natural Sexual Impulse, Normal Sexual Habits and Propagation, Together with Sexual Physiology and Hygiene*, 6th ed. (St. Louis: C. V. Mosby, 1923), 56–57.

108. A. K. Gardner, "The Hygiene of the Sewing Machine," *American Medical Times* 1 (1860): 420–21, 435–37; "Influence of Sewing Machine on Female Health," *New Orleans Medical and Surgical Journal* 20 (November 1867): 359–60; J. Langdon H. Down, "On the Influence of the Sewing Machine on Female Health," *British Medical Journal* 1 (1867): 26–27; Charles H. Hendricks, "The Sewing Machine Problem as Seen through the Pages of the *American Journal of Obstetrics and Diseases of Women and Children*, 1868–1873," *Obstetrics and Gynecology* 26 (1965): 453–54; Goodell, *Lessons in Gynecology*, 548; Horatio Robinson Storer, *Female Hygiene: A Lecture Delivered at Sacramento and San Francisco, by Request of the State Board of Health of California* (Boston: James Campbell, 1872); and Karen Offen, "'Powered by a Woman's Foot': A Documentary Introduction to the Sexual Politics of the Sewing Machine in Nineteenth-Century France," *Women's Studies International Forum* 11, no. 2 (1988): 93–101.

109. Robert Latou Dickinson, "Bicycling for Women from the Standpoint of the Gynecologist," *American Journal of Obstetrics and Diseases of Women and Children* 31, no. 1 (1895): 24–37.

110. W. E. Fitch, "Bicycle Riding: Its Moral Effect upon Young Girls and Its Relation to Diseases of Women," *Georgia Journal of Medicine and Surgery* 4 (1899): 156; quoted in Haller and Haller, *Physician and Sexuality in Victorian America*, 185.

111. Robert William Taylor, *A Practical Treatise on Sexual Disorders of the Male and Female*, 3d ed. (Philadelphia: Lea Brothers, 1905), 413.

112. Russell Thacher Trall, *Pathology of the Reproductive Organs: Embracing All Forms of Sexual Disorder* (Boston: B. Emerson, 1863), 139, 144.

113. Alphonso David Rockwell, *The Medical and Surgical Uses of Electricity*, new ed. (New York: E. B. Treat, 1903), 635; see also Keystone Electric Company, *Illustrated Catalogue*, 63. On vibratory helmets, "Vibratory Therapeutics," *Scientific American* 67 (October 22, 1892): 265, shows a helmet invented by Gilles de la Tourette at the Salpêtrière. One of John Harvey Kellogg's biographers credits his subject with inventing the jolting chair as well as Taylor's "Manipulator," but the indefatigable Kellogg was in fact a John-Harvey-Come-Lately where therapeutic shaking of patients was concerned; see Richard W. Schwarz, *John Harvey Kellogg, MD* (Nashville: Southern Publishing Association, [ca. 1970]), 124.

114. "An Electrical Rocking Chair," *Scientific American* 68 (May 6, 1893): 276. On the rocking chair as sex gadget, see Bernard Rudofsky, *Now I Lay Me Down to Eat: Notes and Footnotes on the Lost Art of Living* (Garden City, N.Y.: Anchor Books, 1980, 86–91).

115. Good Health Publishing Company, *Twentieth Century Therapeutic Appliances* (Battle Creek, Mich.: Good Health, 1909), 64–73.

116. Joseph Mortimer Granville, *Nerve-Vibration and Excitation as Agents in the Treatment of Functional Disorders and Organic Disease* (London: J. and A. Churchill, 1883), 38, 57.

117. Friedrich Eduard Bilz, *The New Natural Method of Healing* (London: A. Bilz, 1898), 1816.

118. Mary Lydia Hastings Arnold Snow, *Mechanical Vibration and Its Therapeutic Application* (New York: Scientific Authors, 1904); Schall and Son, *Electro-medical Instruments and Their Management*, 17th ed. (London: Schall and Son, 1925), 100.

119. Alfred Levertin, *Dr. G. Zander's Medico-mechanical Gymnastics: Its Method, Importance and Applications* (Stockholm: P. A. Norstedt, 1893); see also Hartvig Nissen, *Swedish Movement and Massage Treatment* (Philadelphia: F. A. Davis, 1890).

120. U.S. Patent Office, *Subject Matter Index of Patents for Inventions Issued by the United States Patent Office from 1790 to 1873* (Washington, D.C.: Government Printing Office, 1874; reprint New York: Arno, 1976), 2:912, patents 86,604 and 122,500; George H. Taylor, "Improvement in Medical Rubbing Apparatus," U.S. Patent 175,202, dated March 21, 1876, application filed May 17, 1875; and "Movement Cure," U.S. Patent 263,625, dated August 29, 1882, application filed June 19, 1882.

121. George Henry Taylor, *Pelvic and Hernial Therapeutics* (New York: J. B. Alden, 1885), 118–33, and Taylor, *Mechanical Aids in the Treatment of Chronic Forms of Disease* (New York: Rodgers, 1893), 75.

122. George Henry Taylor, *Health for Women* (New York: John B. Alden, 1883), 198.

123. Rockwell, *Medical and Surgical Uses of Electricity*, 635, 641.

124. Mortimer Granville, *Nerve-Vibration*, 57.

125. The Bakken Library and Museum of Electricity in Life has a Weiss vibrator (accession no. 82.100) tentatively dated ca. 1925, which somewhat resembles Mortimer Granville's 1886 illustration. The Bakken artifact has a vibrating coil with bar and probe accessories operating on internal dry cell batteries; the older model shown in Mortimer Granville's book has a separate and apparently larger battery.

126. Snow, *Mechanical Vibration*, 1904 and 1912 editions; see also Monell, *System of Instruction in X-Ray Methods*, 589–99.

127. Melanchthon R. Waggoner, *The Note Book of an Electro-therapist* (Chicago: McIntosh Electrical, 1923), 127; Maurice Fiescher Pilgrim, *Mechanical Vibratory Stimulation; Its Theory and Application in the Treatments of Disease* (New York: Lawrence Press, [ca. 1903]), 139–40; Edward B. Lent, *Being Done Good: Comments on the Advance Made by Medical Science during the Past 5,500 Years in the Treatment of Rheumatism* (Brooklyn, N.Y.: Brooklyn Eagle Press, 1904), 225; Mary Cushman Rice, *Electricity in Gynecology* (Chicago: Laing, 1909), 137–38; and Franklin Benjamin Gottschalk, *Static Electricity, X-Ray and Electro-vibration: Their Therapeutic Application* (Chicago: Eisele, 1903), 137–40.

128. Monica Krippner, *The Quality of Mercy: Women at War, Serbia 1915–1918* (London: David and Charles, 1980), 182. The Shelton vibrator was "chosen by the British Commission for use in Allied Hospitals." See also Shelton Electric Company, *The Relief of Pain and the Treatment of Disease by Vibration: Shelton Electric Vibrator* (New York: Shelton Electric, 1917; facsimile reprint San Francisco: Down There Press, 1981), 17.

129. Wallian, *Rhythmotherapy*, 84–85, 185. For fluid-cushion vibratodes, see Sam J. Gorman Company (Chicago), *The Physician's Vibragenitant* (Chicago: Sam J. Gorman, 1905), and the same company's *Electro Therapeutic Apparatus* (Chicago: Sam J. Gorman, [ca. 1912]).

130. Alfred Dale Covey, *Profitable Office Specialities* (Detroit: Physicians Supply Company, 1912), 18.

131. Wappler Electric Manufacturing Company, *Wappler Cautery and Light Apparatus and Accessories* (New York: Wappler Electric Manufacturing, 1914), 7, 42–43, and Manhattan Electrical Supply Company, *Catalogue Twenty-six: Something Electrical for Everybody* (New York: MESCO, n.d.).

132. Vibrator Instrument Company, *The Chattanooga Vibrator* (Chattanooga, Tenn.: Vibrator Instrument, [ca. 1904]), 3, 26. See also Vibrator Instrument Company, *A Treatise on Vibration and Mechanical Stimulation* (Chattanooga, Tenn.: Vibrator Instrument, 1902).

133. Vibrator Instrument Company, Clinical Department, *A Course on Mechanical Vibratory Stimulation* (New York: Vibrator Instrument, 1903), 8, 22.

134. Franklin Benjamin Gottschalk, *Practical Electro-therapeutics, with a Special Section on Vibratory Stimulation* (Hammond, Ind.: F. S. Betz, 1903), 45, 118.

135. Anthony Matijaca, *Principles of Electro-medicine, Electro-surgery and Radiology* (Tangerine, Fla.: Benedict Lust, 1917), 134. As tempting as it is to speculate, I doubt there is any significance to the name of the publisher, a reputable producer of medical works at the turn of this century.

136. Samuel Spencer Wallian, "The Undulatory Theory in Therapeutics . . . First Paper," *Medical Brief*, May 1905.

137. Samuel Spencer Wallian, "The Undulatory Theory in Therapeutics . . . Second Paper," *Medical Brief*, June 1905.

138. D. T. Smith, *Vibration and Life* (Boston: Richard G. Badger, Gorham Press, 1912).

139. Mortimer Granville, *Nerve-Vibration*, 14, 20.

140. Golden Manufacturing Company, *Vibration: Nature's Great Underlying Force for Health, Strength and Beauty* (Detroit, Mich.: Golden Manufacturing, 1914), unpaged; see also Professor Rohrer's Institute of Beauty Culture, *Rohrer's Illustrated Book on Scientific Modern Beauty Culture* (New York: Professor Rohrer's Institute, 1924), 39–41, and [William Meyer], *The Cosmetiste*, 9th ed. (Chicago: William Meyer, 1936), 179–91. For the vibrator in European beauty salons, see Magnus Hirschfeld and Richard Linsert, *Liebes Mittel* (Berlin: Man, 1930), 554, and "Kosmetik," in *Bilder-Lexikon Kulturgeschichte*, vol. 1 (Vienna: Verlag für Kulturforschung, 1928), 553–54.

141. Good Health, *Twentieth Century Therapeutic Appliances*, 64.

142. Sigvard Strandh, *A History of the Machine* (New York: A. and W., 1979), 225–26; Malcolm MacLaren, *The Rise of the Electrical Industry during the Nineteenth Century* (Princeton: Princeton University Press, 1943), 91, 96; Earl Lifshey, *The Housewares Story* (Chicago: National Housewares Manufacturers Association, 1973), 281; Helen Lamborn, "Electricity for Domestic Uses," *Harper's Bazaar* 44 (April 1910): 285; and "White Magic: Facts You Want to Know about It," *Modern Priscilla*, February 1923, 55–57. On fans and irons, see Siegfried Giedion, *Mechanization Takes Command* (New York: Oxford University Press, 1948), 558–59, 572–73.

143. "Neuralgia, Headache, Wrinkles. The Vibratile Electric Massage," Hutches and Company (Chicago), advertisement in *McClure's Magazine*, March 1899, 64e.

144. "Your Hands Properly Used are all You Need to Earn $3000 to $5000 a Year," American College of Mechano-therapy (Chicago), advertisement in *Men and Women*, April 1910, inside front cover.

145. "This Marvelous Health Vibrator for Man, Woman and Child. Relieves All Suffering. Cures Disease," Lambert Snyder Company (New York), advertisement in *Modern Women* 11, no. 5 (1907): 170.

146. "TO WOMEN I address my message of health and beauty," Bebout Vibrator Company (St. Louis, Mo.), advertisement in *National Home Journal*, April 1908, 17.

147. "Hydro-Massage for the Complexion. For the Scalp. For the Nerves." Warner Motor Company, Inc. (New York), advertisement in *Modern Women* 11, no. 1 (1906): 190.

148. "Corbin Vacuo-Masseur, for Facial Massage. A Flesh Builder. Removes Wrinkles and Other Blemishes," Becton, Dickinson and Company (Rutherford, N.J.), advertisement in *Woman's Home Companion* 36 (May 1909): 57.

149. "Agents! Drop Dead Ones! Awake! Grab this new invention! The 20th century wonder, Blackstone Water Power Vacuum Massage Machine," Blackstone Manufacturing Company (Toledo, Ohio), advertisement in *Hearst's*, April 1916, 327.

150. "If Your Beauty is Marred by a serious or a slight blemish . . . ," Mahler Electrical Apparatus (Providence, R.I.), advertisement in *Bohemian*, December 1909, 817.

151. "Electricity the Renewer of Youth," *Review of Reviews* 37 (June 1908): 732–33, and Mildred Maddocks, "Electricity Your Summer Servant," *Good Housekeeping* 63 (July 1916): 126.

152. American Vibrator Company, *Vibratory Stimulation: The American Vibrator* (St. Louis, Mo.: American Vibrator, [ca. 1906]), 1, 8; and American Vibrator Company (St. Louis, Mo.), "Massage is as old as the hills—it's [*sic*] value as an alleviating, curative, and beautifying agent is endorsed by all reputable physicians," advertisement in *Woman's Home Companion*, April 1906, 42.

153. Swedish Vibrator Company (Chicago), "Wanted. Agents and salesmen. Sell the Swedish vibrator," advertisement in *Modern Priscilla*, April 1913, 60.

154. Monarch Vibrator Company (Jackson, Mich.), "Sent on approval . . . Monarch Electric Massage Vibrator," advertisement in *Hearst's Magazine*, February 1916, 159.

155. William Lee Howard, *Sex Problems in Worry and Work* (New York: Edward J. Clode, 1915). Howard was also the author of *Plain Facts on Sex Hygiene* (1910) and *Facts for the Married* (1912), both also published by Edward J. Clode.

156. "The Home Electrical," in *A General Electric Scrapbook History with Commentary* ([Schenectady, N.Y.?]: General Electric, 1953).

157. J. J. Duck Company, *Anything Electrical* (Toledo, Ohio: J. J. Duck, 1912), 162, 278. Track was not included in the price of the train set.

158. Sears, Roebuck and Company, *Electrical Goods: Everything Electrical for Home, Office, Factory and Shop* (Chicago: Sears, Roebuck, 1918), 4, 8, 9.

159. Star Home Electric Massage Vibrators, "A Gift that Will *Keep* Her Young and Pretty," advertisement in *Hearst's International*, December 1921, 82, and "Such Delightful Companions!" advertisement, 1922, reproduced in *Those Were the Good Old Days*, ed. Edgar R. Jones (New York: Simon and Schuster, 1959), 60.

160. "Electra" [pseud.], "Useful Hints for the Homemaker," *Electrical Age for Women* (Glasgow) 2, no. 7 (1932): 275. See also advertisement for "Pneumatic massage pulsator" inside front cover of the same issue.

161. Lindstrom Smith Company (Chicago), "Vibration is Life!" advertisement in *Technical World*, ca. 1902, unpaged advertising section.

162. David J. Pivar, *Purity Crusade: Sexual Morality and Social Control, 1868–1900* (Westport, Conn.: Greenwood Press, 1973), 110–17.

163. Lindstrom Smith Company (Chicago), "Send for our Free Book . . . White Cross Electric Vibrator," advertisement in *Home Needlework Magazine*, October 1908, 479, and *National Home Journal*, April 1909, 24.

164. Lindstrom Smith Company (Chicago), "Vibration is Life . . . White Cross Electric Vibrator," advertisement in *Modern Priscilla*, December 1910, 27. See also "Beauty is Yours," advertisement in *Needlecraft*, September 1912, 23, and in the *American Magazine* 75, no. 2 (1912): 118.

165. Lindstrom Smith Company (Chicago), "Enjoy Life! Get all you can out of it," advertisement for the White Cross Vibrator in the *American Magazine* 75, no. 3 (1913): 118.

166. Lindstrom Smith Company (Chicago), "Power for you," advertisement for the White Cross Vibrator in *American Magazine* 75, no. 7 (1913): 127; see also advertisements in *Hearst's Magazine*, January 1916, 67; February 1916, 154; April 1916, 329; and June 1916, 473. In the April 1916 issue, an advertisement for William H. Walling's *Sexology* (Philadelphia: Puritan, 1912) appears on the same page.

167. Lindstrom and Company (Chicago), "Stop that Pain!" advertisement for the Elco Electric Health Generator, in *Popular Mechanics*, December 1928, unpaged advertising section.

168. See, for example, Frederick's of Hollywood, *Get It Now and Save!* catalog 74, vol. 31, no. 211 (1977). Robert J. Francoeur gives 1966 as the date when "Plastic, battery-power vibrators became popular in drugstores and supermarkets." See Francoeur, *Becoming a Sexual Person* (New York: John Wiley, 1982), 37.

169. Niresk Industries of Chicago seems to have been an important producer of massagers at this period, as was Spot Reducer of Newark, New Jersey. See advertisements in *Workbasket* 16, no. 6 (1951): 23; 17, no. 3 (1951): 33; 18, no. 2 (1952): 70; 22, no. 11 (August 1957): 3; 23, no. 12 (September 1958): 91, 93; 24, no. 1 (October 1958): 95; and 24, no. 3 (December 1958): 47.

170. Roger Blake, *Sex Gadgets* (Cleveland: Century Books, 1968), 33–34, 46.

171. Albert Ellis, *If This Be Sexual Heresy* (New York: Lyle Stuart, 1963), 136.

172. Paul Tabori, *The Humor and Technology of Sex* (New York: Julian Press, 1969), 444.

173. Blake, *Sex Gadgets*, 121; Mimi Swartz, "For the Woman Who Has Almost Everything," *Esquire*, July 1980, 56–63; and Helen Singer Kaplan, "The Vibrator: A Misunderstood Machine," *Redbook*, May 1984, 34.

174. Helen Singer Kaplan, *The New Sex Therapy* (New York: Brunner-Mazel, 1974), 388–89.

175. See, for examples, Kaplan, *New Sex Therapy*, 361–90, esp. 388–89, and Edward Dengrove, "The Mechanotherapy of Sexual Disorders," *Journal of Sex Research* 7, no. 1 (1971): 5–9. Dengrove also reported that some of his patients achieved satisfactory results with a soft-bristle electric toothbrush.

176. Dengrove, "Mechanotherapy of Sexual Disorders," 7–8.

177. Susan Strasser, *Never Done: A History of American Housework* (New York: Pantheon Books, 1982), 306.

Chapter 5 Revising the Androcentric Model

1. Alexander Lowen, *Love and Orgasm* (New York: Macmillan, 1965), 216.

2. Sophie Lazarsfeld, *Woman's Experience of the Male* (London: Encyclopedic Press, 1967), 105.

3. A summary and overview of this subject appear in Anne McClintock's special section on the sex trade in *Social Text,* no. 37 (winter 1993). See especially McClintock's introduction, 1–10.

4. Mills says that "in Briquet's often-quoted 1000 cases of hysteria, 50 only occurred in men." See Charles K. Mills, "Hysteria," in *A System of Practical Medicine*, vol. 5, *Diseases of the Nervous System*, ed. William Pepper and Louis Starr (Philadelphia: Lea Brothers, 1886), 215.

5. Helen Singer Kaplan and Erica Sucher, "Women's Sexual Response," in *Women's Sexual Experience: Explorations of the Dark Continent*, ed. Martha Kirkpatrick (New York: Plenum Press, 1982), 9–12.

6. Wilhelm Reich, *The Function of the Orgasm* (New York: Farrar, Straus and Giroux, 1973), 95–116.

7. Feminist criticism of the androcentric model has appeared in the works of professionals such as Helen Kaplan and in popular publications such as *Our Bodies, Ourselves*. In Boston Women's Health Book Collective, *The New Our Bodies, Ourselves* (New York: Simon and Schuster, 1984), the authors observe that "most people define sex mainly in terms of intercourse, a form of lovemaking which is often well suited to men's orgasm and pleasure but is not necessarily well suited to ours" (185).

8. Carole S. Vance, "Gender Systems, Ideology and Sex Research," in *Powers of Desire: The Politics of Sexuality*, ed. Ann Snitow, Christine Stansell, and Sharon Thompson (New York: Monthly Review Press, 1983), 373–78.

9. Seymour Fisher, *The Female Orgasm: Psychology, Physiology, Fantasy* (New York: Basic Books, 1973), 297, 410.

10. Jeanne Warner, "Physical and Affective Dimensions of Peak of Female Sexual Response and the Relationship to Self-Reported Orgasm," in *International Research in Sexology: Selected Papers from the Fifth World Congress*, ed. Harold Lief and Zwi Hoch (New York: Praeger, 1984), 94.

11. Frank S. Caprio, *The Adequate Male* (New York: Medical Research Press, 1952), 70.

12. David Reuben, despite his penetrationist views on orgasm during coitus, takes a pro-woman stance on this issue. See *Any Woman Can! Love and Sexual Fulfillment for the Single, Widowed, Divorced . . . and Married* (New York: D. McKay, 1971), 25–56.

13. Frank S. Caprio, *The Sexually Adequate Female* (New York: Medical Research Press, 1953), 77, 83–187. See esp. 94 on the "hysterical personality."

14. There are illustrations of this problem among the anecdotes reported in Linda Wolfe, *The Cosmo Report* (New York: Arbor House, 1981), 121–50.

15. Auguste Debay, *Hygiène du mariage* (Paris: Moquet, 1848).

16. Celia Roberts, Susan Kippax, Catherine Waldby, and June Crawford, "Faking It: The Story of 'Ohh!'" *Women's Studies International Forum* 18, nos. 5–6 (1995): 523–25, 528. There is an amusing reference to this behavior in the restaurant scene of the movie *When Harry Met Sally*.

17. Michael Segell, "Great Performances," *Esquire*, January 1996, 30.

18. Glen Freyer, "What Do Men Know, or Think They Know, about the Female Orgasm?" *Glamour* 93, no. 4 (1995): 128.

19. For a subjective account of the difficulty of speaking the truth in these situations, see Molly Peacock's poem "Have You Ever Faked an Orgasm?" *Paris Review* 36, no. 130 (1994): 255.

20. Dolores Haze, "Faking It," *Mademoiselle* 100, no. 1 (1994): 125. Haze points out that "while women fake to save their mates' feelings, men fake to save face." Faking, of course, is much less common among men.

21. Carol Tavris and Susan Sadd, *The Redbook Report on Female Sexuality* (New York: Delacorte, 1977), 79.

22. Robert T. Francoeur, *Becoming a Sexual Person* (New York: John Wiley, 1982), 588.

23. Stephanie Alexander, "Was It Good for You Too?" *Cosmopolitan* 218, no. 5 (1995): 80.

24. "Changing Sexuality in a Changing Society: The Hite Reports," in Organization of American Historians and National Council on Public History, 1986 *Program* (New York: OAH, 1986), 50.

25. This seems to be true even in visual representations of my research. See, for example, John Orentlicher's video, *Misaligned Shafts* (Syracuse, N.Y.: Syracuse University Art Department, 1989).

26. Edward Kelly, "A New Image for the Naughty Dildo?" *Journal of Popular Culture* 7, no. 4 (1974): 808.

27. A version of this appears in Roz Warren's *Glibquips: Funny Words by Funny Women* (Freedom, Calif.: Crossing Press, 1994), 103.

28. Michael Adas, *Machines as the Measure of Men: Science, Technology and Ideologies of Western Dominance* (Ithaca: Cornell University Press, 1989).

29. Dianne Grosskopf, *Sex and the Married Woman* (New York: Simon and Schuster, 1983), 119.

30. Melvin Kranzberg, "Technology and History: 'Kranzberg's Laws,'" *Technology and Culture* 27, no. 3 (1986): 545.

Note on Sources

In preparing this book I consulted over five hundred works. Readers will be relieved to learn that I do not propose to describe them all but only intend to sketch the outlines of my own journey through the various literatures that bear on the histories of medicine, technology, and sexuality. I am often asked if I did not have great difficulty locating material. It is certainly true that the secondary literature of vibrators is very small, but I was virtually buried in primary material on medicine and sexuality. After more than ten years dedicated to tracking down and reading obscure (and not so obscure) references, I still feel that I have barely chipped the surface of the vast iceberg of Western medical literature. The pre-1750 strata of this imposing mass are submerged in untranslated medical Latin, a language for which even a former classics major like me is unprepared. Arnaldus of Villanova (d. 1311) and Hermann Boerhaave (1668–1738) certainly wrote in Latin, but theirs is not the language of Virgil and Cicero.

In selecting from this vast body of work, I have attempted to survey the Who's Whos of hysteria included in major modern works on the subject, particularly Ilsa Veith's *Hysteria: The History of a Disease* (1965), George Wesley's *History of Hysteria* (1979), and Phillip Slavney's *Perspectives on "Hysteria"* (1990), plus a few items mentioned by Havelock Ellis. Audrey Eccles provides valuable background on some of the gynecological sources in her *Obstetrics and Gynaecology in Tudor and Stuart England* (1982). Most of the medical luminaries in the hysteria-gynecology galaxy are better known for other contributions: Aretaeus Cappodox, Soranus, Celsus, Avicenna, Rhazes, Rivière, Boerhaave, Harvey, Cullen, Galen, Haller, Zacuto, Paré, Mandeville, Paracelsus, Pinel, Rodrigues de Castro, and Sydenham are all names to reckon with in medical history. There are, however, a great many lesser lights who wrote on hysteria and other disorders of women but whose works are available only in large libraries and only in Latin. *Caveat lector:* only the unabridged *Oxford Latin Dictionary* will avail with the vocabulary, and even this resource is sometimes found wanting.

As recently as fifteen years ago it was difficult to find secondary sources on the history of sexuality, but now there is a large and growing literature to guide the scholar. I found John D'Emilio and Estelle Freedman's *Intimate Matters: A History of Sexuality in America* (1988) and Thomas Laqueur's *Making Sex: Body and Gender from the Greeks to Freud* (1990) particularly useful. John S. Haller and Robin Haller's *The Physician and Sexuality in Victorian America* (1973) provides an overview of many of the issues I have addressed in detail here. Most historians will have seen Peter Gay's monumental *The Bourgeois Experience: Victoria to Freud* (1984) and Michel Foucault's *History of Sexuality* (1978). Earlier European history is ably addressed in Danielle Jacquart and Claude Thomasset's *Sexuality and Medicine in the Middle Ages* (1988). For medical advice literature and gynecological works in the United States, I can warmly recommend Nancy Sahli's *Women and Sexuality in America: A Bibliography* (1984).

The subject of masturbation is mentioned in book-length secondary sources on the history of sexuality, but serious scholars of the subject will want to start with a few important articles (one dare not call them "seminal"): Vern Bullough's article on technology for preventing masturbation in the October 1987 issue of *Technology and Culture;* Donald Greydanus's "Masturbation: Historic Perspective," in the *New York State Journal of Medicine* for November 1980; E. H. Hare's "Masturbatory Insanity: The History of an Idea," in the *Journal of Mental Science*, vol. 108 (1962); and Robert H. MacDonald's "The Frightful Consequences of Onanism: Notes on the History of a Delusion," in the *Journal of the History of Ideas*, July–September 1967.

Hydrotherapy is addressed in an eclectic combination of primary and secondary sources. Henri Scoutetten (1799–1871), for example, wrote a book called *De l'eau* (1843), which contains nothing particularly original about hydriatic treatments but includes a bibliography of all works on the subject before his time so comprehensive that I could locate fewer than half of them in modern union lists such the Library of Congress's *Pre-1956 Imprints*. Hundreds of books were written on hydrotherapy between ancient times and the mid-nineteenth century. Much of this material is scattered through European libraries. There are a few good secondary sources on hydrotherapy and a great many popular histories. I recommend Susan Cayleff's dissertation "Wash and Be Healed: The Nineteenth-Century Water-Cure Movement, 1840–1900" (1983); Jane Donegan's *Hydropathic Highway to Health: Women and Water-Cure in Antebellum America* (1986); and Patricia Spain Ward's *Simon Baruch: Rebel in the Ranks of Medicine, 1840–1921* (1994) for readers who wish to gain an overview of the personalities and institutions of the hydropathic and hydrotherapeutic world. I found many of the primary sources I was looking for on this subject in the Saratoga Room collection of the Saratoga (New York) Public Library and at the Saratoga County Historical Society in nearby Ballston Spa.

As I explained in the preface, this book could not have been written without the resources of the Bakken Library in Minneapolis, which holds artifact and document collections on every conceivable (and inconceivable) aspect of electricity in the life sciences, including disreputable and usually ephemeral advertising material for long-vanished medical devices. I found many of the more general medical and scientific works at the National Library of Medicine and in the Kroch Library and Archives of Cornell University, both well-known repositories. The Kinsey Institute at Indiana University has important and comprehensive print, motion picture, and photographic documentation of the history of sexuality, including popular works rarely to be found in other libraries, even very large ones. Historians of medicine seeking an excuse to spend time in Paris could hardly do better than to plan a research trip to the Charcot Library of the Salpêtrière. The collections and the environment are both rich and fascinating.

Bibliographic access to the popular periodicals I have cited here is very difficult. The magazines themselves are hard to find and, when found, are often brittle, discolored, and crumbling because they were originally produced on pulp paper, the problem conservators call "inherent vice." They are rarely or never indexed; the further downmarket one explores in household magazines, the less likely the publication is to be listed in a respectable index like the *Reader's Guide*. The New York Public Library and the Library of Congress both have excellent but crumbling collections of such periodicals as the *American Magazine*, *National Home Journal*, *Men and Women*, *Woman's Home Companion*, *Cosmopolitan*, *Bohemian*, *Hearst's*, *Modern Woman*, *Home Needlework*, *Modern Priscilla*, and *Good Stories*. Some have been microfilmed.

Index

Books in the New Series

1. *The American Railroad Passenger Car* John H. White Jr.
2. *Neptune's Gift: A History of Common Salt* Robert P. Multhauf
3. *Electricity before Nationalisation: A Study of the Development of the Electricity Supply Industry in Britain to 1948* Leslie Hannah
4. *Alexander Holley and the Makers of Steel* Jeanne McHugh
5. *The Origins of the Turbojet Revolution* Edward W. Constant
6. *Engineers, Managers, and Politicians: The First Fifteen Years of Nationalised Electricity Supply in Britain* Leslie Hannah
7. *Stronger Than a Hundred Men: A History of the Vertical Water Wheel* Terry S. Reynolds
8. *Authority, Liberty, and Automatic Machinery in Early Modern Europe* Otto Mayr
9. *Inventing American Broadcasting, 1899–1922* Susan J. Douglas
10. *Edison and the Business of Innovation* Andre Millard
11. *What Engineers Know and How They Know It: Analytical Studies from Aeronautical History* Walter G. Vincenti
12. *Alexanderson: Pioneer in American Electrical Engineering* James E. Brittain
13. *Steinmetz: Engineer and Socialist* Ronald R. Kline
14. *From Machine Shop to Industrial Laboratory: Telegraphy and the Changing Context of American Invention, 1830–1920* Paul Israel

15. *The Course of Industrial Decline: The Boott Cotton Mills of Lowell, Massachusetts, 1835–1955* Lawrence F. Gross

16. *High Performance: The Culture and Technology of Drag Racing, 1950–1990* Robert C. Post

17. *A Nation of Steel: The Making of Modern America, 1865–1925* Thomas J. Misa

18. *Transforming Computer Technology: Information Processing for the Pentagon, 1962–1986* Arthur L. Norberg and Judy E. O'Neill, with contributions by Kerry Freedman

19. *American Iron, 1607–1900* Robert B. Gordon

20. *All the Modern Conveniences: American Household Plumbing, 1840–1890* Maureen Ogle

21. *The Machine in the Nursery: Incubator Technology and the Origins of Newborn Intensive Care* Jeffrey P. Baker

22. *Weapons and Warfare in Renaissance Europe: Gunpowder, Technology, and Tactics* Bert S. Hall

23. *Manmade Weather: Air Conditioning in the United States, 1900–1960* Gail Cooper

24. *The Technology of Orgasm: "Hysteria," the Vibrator, and Women's Sexual Satisfaction* Rachel P. Maines

Library of Congress Cataloging-in-Publication Data

Maines, Rachel P.
The technology of orgasm : "hysteria," the vibrator, and women's sexual satisfaction / Rachel P. Maines.
p. cm. — (Johns Hopkins studies in the history of technology ; new ser., no. 24)
Includes bibliographical references and index.
ISBN 0-8018-5941-7 (alk. paper)
1. Women—Sexual behavior—History. 2. Female orgasm—History.
3. Anorgasmy—History. 4. Masturbation—History. 5. Vibrators—History.
I. Title. II. Series.
HQ29.M35 1998
306.7'082'09—dc21 98-20213
CIP